Gretel —

Thank you for your encouragement to write a book — years ago — Thank you for planting the seed —

CR Mancerk—
Jami

Disclaimer
The information presented herein is offered only for informational and educational purposes and is not a substitute for the professional judgment of a medical professional. We strongly recommend that you receive professional medical advice before you perform any techniques, poses, postures or routines presented in this book. The reader and viewer of the information presented in this publication assumes all risks when using the information provided herein. Any information provided in this publication is not intended as a replacement for professional consultations with qualified practitioners. If this publication provides health-related or medical information, no such information provided by this book is intended to treat or cure any disease or to offer any specific diagnosis to any individual as we do not give medical advice, nor do we provide medical or diagnostic services.

All rights reserved. No part of this publication may be reproduced, stored in a retrieval system, or transmitted in any form or by any means, electronic, mechanical, photocopying, recording or otherwise, without the prior permission in writing of the publisher, except in the case of brief quotations embodied in a book review.

Therapeutic Answers
to Common Yoga Pose Questions
2nd Print

For yoga students & teachers

who have a basic understanding of yoga and their bodies

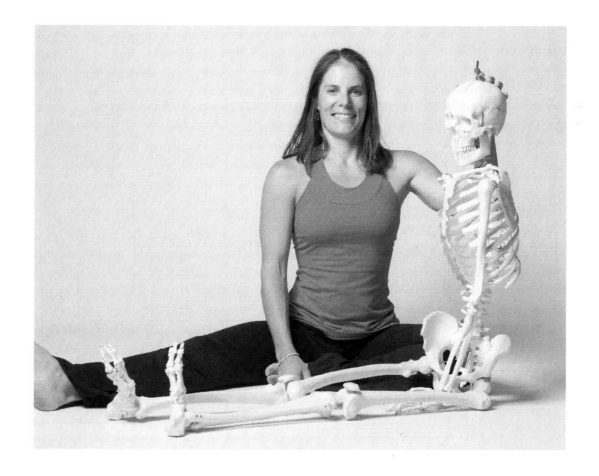

Jaimie Perkunas
DPT, e-RYT

Copyright © Jaimie Perkunas, 2016

Foreword

I have been a student of Jaimie Perkunas for about two years. Like many of her yoga students, I have an orthopedic history that restricted my range of motion pretty severely. I was pretty bionic when I met Jaimie; a total replacement of both hips around fifteen years earlier, and total replacement of both shoulders three years ago. Perhaps just as traumatic, I spent many years seated at a desk, working seventy hours per week. The result of all of this was that, while I was active, playing tennis regularly, practicing tai chi chuan and going to the gym, I was very inflexible. My movement was restricted, and I injured myself pretty frequently. I came to yoga, and to Jaimie, to see what improvement was possible. I was very concerned about the possibility of injury, and took some comfort in the fact that she was a physical therapist.

The results, two years in, have pleased me beyond my most generous expectations. I am far more mobile than I was when I started. Simple things that were difficult at the start—such as lowering to one knee from a standing position—I now do without hesitation. Having greatly expanded my range of motion and strength, I move better, injure myself less and am pain free.

Like anyone active at my age (I'm sixty five), I occasionally strain a muscle or overwork a tendon, and see Jaimie for individual instruction. It is those times when I most appreciate how physical therapy and yoga complement each other. When you have had as much surgery as I have, you get to do a lot of physical therapy. Jaimie's approach, using yoga poses as therapy, has proven to be more effective, and far faster, than traditional PT. Yoga seems a far more comprehensive way to recover from injury than the usual physical therapy modalities. It is also a lot more fun to do.

This book contains Jaimie's answers to questions from her students, clients and others. Her answers show the anatomy-based approach that she takes to yoga, and to its use in healing. There is a great deal of information here of value for all yoga practitioners, whether or not they are limited in motion by injury or surgery. Her substantial knowledge of the human body informs and enriches yoga practice for everyone. I hope it does for you what it has done for me.

Paul Winick
Tucson, Arizona
March 2016

Dedication

To all my students and clients, who continue to ask me to grow and learn.

Acknowledgements

To my visionary husband who encouraged me to share my knowledge as a physical therapist with my experiences with yoga.

To my Dad, who planted the seed long ago that I would be a yoga teacher.

To my Mom, who has inspired me write this book with her first-hand experiences of yoga challenges.

To Jade Beall for her professional photos throughout the book, and Tom Beall for being my alignment coach during the photo shoot.

To Rebecca Grad for her beautiful drawings of anatomy.

To Barb Duro for editing my newsletters and this book.

To Amanda Beekhuizen for designing and editing this book.

To Gina Rooney for editing this book.

To all my yoga teachers: Rachel Krentzman, Bruce Bowditch, Darren Rhodes, and Christina Sell.

To my colleagues and mentors: Staffan Elgelid, Matthew Taylor, Shelley Prosko, Neil Pearson, Lisa Holland, and the Bridgebuilder community.

To the many students who have asked questions and trusted me to help you with your healing and recovery.

To all my friends near and far, who have encouraged me along the way: Tanya, Rebecca, Gina, and many more.

Table of Contents

Introduction	1
Lower body	**3**
Bunions	4
Stretching arches	11
Weak ankles	16
Nerve flossing	22
Knocked knee	25
Baker's Cyst	28
Standing forward fold	29
Standing quad stretch	35
IT band	39
Stretching after pregnancy	43
Sciatica	45
Piriformis syndrome	47
Three ways to address muscle imbalance	52
Hip Replacement	56
Hamstrings/adductor strain and strengthening	66
Hip flexor	74
Upper Body	**77**
Carpal tunnel	78
Tennis and golfer's elbow	83
Upper body nerve flossing	87
Shoulders	93
Shoulder blade stability	103

Wild thing	110
Backbends: bridge and wheel	114
Posture/spine	**119**
TMJ	120
Pain with psoas release	124
Heat vs. ice	128
Posture: Side-lying, seated, and standing	130
Spinal fusion	136
Alternative to inversion table	138
Yin yoga	140
Travel techniques	142
Afterword	151

Introduction

I started my first yoga and physical therapy business in 2011, a month after completing my 200-hour yoga teacher training. During the training, I was asked to teach two hours of anatomy to the trainees since I had been a practicing physical therapist for five years. It was at that point when I realized I had something unique to offer to my yoga community. I am very interested in educating yoga teachers and students about anatomy, biomechanics, and injury prevention. I am particularly interested in assuring that yoga continues to be a safe practice for all students, including those with injury, history of past surgeries, or limitations in range of motion or strength.

Within two years of starting my business I started a monthly newsletter which included a section for Q&A's. I have been writing a monthly newsletter and answering questions for the last three and a half years and wanted to put these therapeutic answers into a common resource. I hope this resource helps to answer your common yoga questions. I would encourage you to contact me with additional questions or need for clarification.

Thank you for your interest in supporting my vision of yoga being appropriate for ANY BODY.

Jaimie Perkunas DPT, e-RYT
Jaimie@yogaistherapy.com
www.yogaistherapy.com

one: the lower body

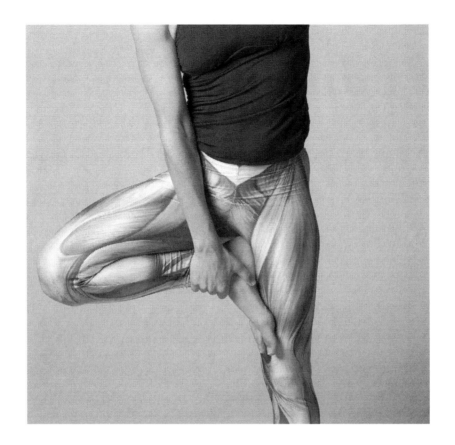

The lower body is the foundation in standing and sitting poses. Although we live our lives with our weight on our lower body whether we are sitting or standing, we are asked in our yoga practices to bring awareness to our lower body with an intention to keep a balance of strength and flexibility. This section will address questions involving the lower body starting from the feet working up to the hips.

Can yoga help bunions?

Yes, I believe yoga can, though there is currently no research yet pointing to yoga as a cure for bunions. However, when I was at my first International Yoga Therapy Conference in Boston in 2013, I spoke with Dr. Loren Fishman about an entry he had in "Yoga as Medicine." I can't remember the exact page, but I remember reading a paragraph where the author referred to Dr. Loren Fishman as having stated that bunions can be improved by strengthening the *abductor hallucis* (*hallucis* is big toe). When I was at the conference I asked him about this in person. He proceeded to remove his dress shoe and dress sock to demonstrate how to activate the *abductor hallucis* (the muscle which pulls the big toe away from the second toe).

My theory is that since muscles move bones, thereby addressing muscle imbalances, a change may occur in the alignment of bones or joints. When a bunion forms it causes additional bone growth on the outside of the first metatarsal (big toe knuckle). This increase in bone growth is likely caused from the *abductor hallucis* tendon being pulled across the lateral (outside) aspect of the joint or from the lateral side of the metatarsal pressing into a tight shoe (narrow toed shoe like high heels or dress shoes). When our bones are subjected to continuous pulling or pressure from pushing or pressing, this can cause increased bone growth which may lead to bunions.

My personal opinion is that if the body can create bone then it can also remove bone once the pressure or pulling is released. I believe that addressing the muscle imbalances in one's big toe muscles can improve and maybe even reduce bunions. Dr. Fishman believes this to be true also and suggested that if I could show improvement with my clients/students that we could do a research study together about this theory.

When a bunion occurs, the big toe is forced over towards the second toe which is called adduction of the big toe. This results in the *abductor hallucis* to be overstretched and weak while the *adductor hallucis* which brings the big into adduction is shortened and tight from the orientation of the big toe being in adduction. I believe massaging and stretching the big toe into abduction will help improve the big toe alignment. Stretching the *adductor hallucis* and strengthening the *abductor hallucis* can improve the muscular imbalance and align the big joint. Bunion formation can cause pain and limitation in big toe extension which is important for push off when walking. Bunions can lead to or be from altered foot orientation while walking, causing the feet to be turned out. The orientation of the feet influences the alignment of the ankles, knees, and hips and may cause pain and discomfort all the way up into the low back and neck. There are some stretching, strengthening, and awareness exercises that can help address the muscle imbalances associated with bunions.

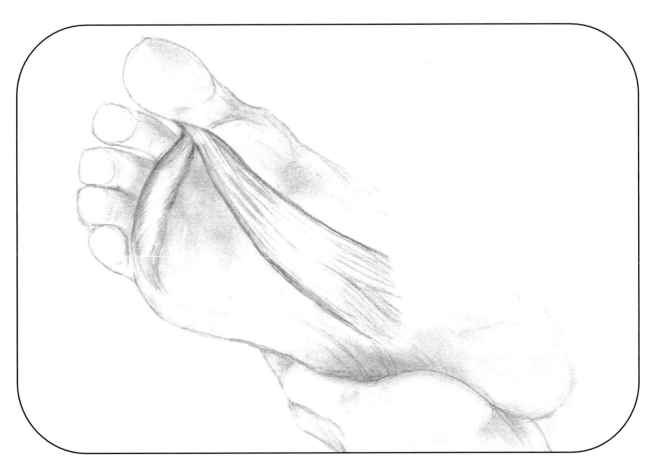

Adductor hallucis of the right foot

Massaging adductor hallucis

Using your fingers or a tennis ball, massage across the ball of your foot from the second toe to the fourth toe.

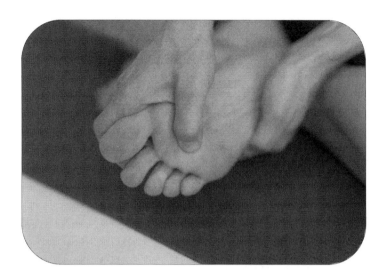

Then massage along the arch of your foot, from the ball of your foot to your heel. Stay in a straight line between your big toe and second toe.

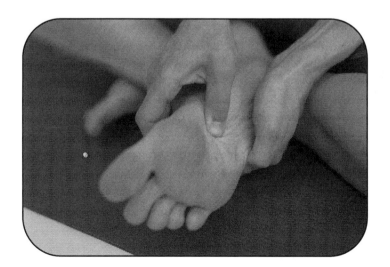

Three Steps to Spreading your Toes

1. Physically pull your big toe away from your second toe. Sustain for ten to fifteen breaths and perform two to three times a day.

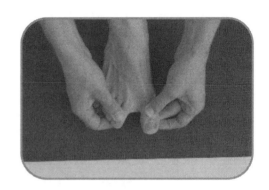

2. Use a tennis ball to help spread your toes. Place a tennis ball on the ball of your foot with your heel on the ground with toes pointing straight ahead.

Press the ball down and spread your toes. Sustain for ten to fifteen breaths. Perform two to three times a day.

3. Perform the exercise again without the tennis ball and try to spread your toes.

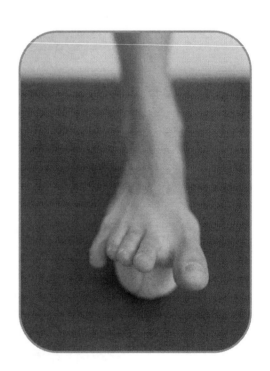

Strengthening your abductor hallucis
in three progressive steps

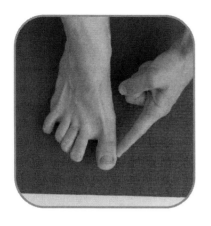

1. Pull your big toe away from your second toe (as above) and then try hold it in position.

2. Press the outside of your big toe into your finger.

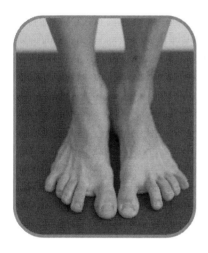

3. In a standing position, press your big toes together (with your heels apart), or use a sticky mat to hold your big toe in place as your pull your heels towards each other.

Perform each of these for five to ten breaths, two to three times a day, and don't forget to wash your hands after doing your exercises.

Perform these exercises and take pictures of your feet before and after six to eight weeks of doing these daily. See if you notice that your bunions have become smaller and if any pain you had has subsided. Bunions take years to develop and may take several months to resolve; be patient and committed.

I find that most of my clients and students who have bunions have limited to no awareness in their feet. Many often believe their bunion development is hereditary and there is nothing they can do. If you would like to make changes to your body, especially in an area so very far away from your eyes, it is essential to bring your awareness to this area on a daily basis.

> *Spread your big toes.*
> *Every time you are in a pose where your feet are together*
> *or even near each other (as in* Tadasana, *chair pose, or*
> *Down Dog), spread your big toes towards each other.*
> *Imagine they are long-lost lovers reaching to be together.*

I have a yoga question for you. I have a student who is also a physical therapist (PT). Last week she asked me a question that I really wasn't sure how to answer. I had them curl their toes under and sit back on their heels to stretch their toes and feet (toe breaker pose). She asked me why I had them doing that, because if you stretch out the arches out of the feet you can never get them back. I was puzzled because I had never heard of that before, and it's something that I see taught often in classes. Is she right? Am I doing something wrong?

I believe it is more good than harmful. There are mixed opinions about stretching fascia. I recently read an article by science writer and massage therapist Paul Ingraham (*Painscience.com* 2016) that argues the two extremes about stretching fascia, one being that fascia *cannot* be stretched and another that fascia can easily be overstretched.

> *Does Fascia Matter?* by Paul Ingraham
> https://www.painscience.com/articles/does-fascia-matter.php

The foot has four layers of muscles and the most superficial (closest to the surface) layer is the fascia. In the "toe-breaker" pose, the flexors of the toes along with the soleus (deep calf muscle) are being stretched. If a person has flat feet (collapsed arches) then I would recommend emphasizing keeping more engagement during the stretch by having them press through the ball of their foot while sustaining the stretch.

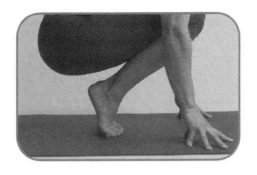 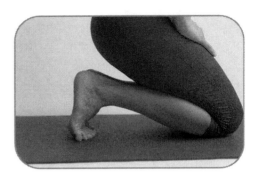

There is a belief that this pose may not be the best for students with flat feet since they have already overstretched their arches. I would recommend keeping engagement through the ball of the foot by coming into a squat and lifting the heels, then slowly shift the weight forward to place the knees on the ground. Keep the toes and ball of foot pressing back like you were pushing yourself forward with the toes. I believe this pose is especially beneficial for the student with high arches or who wears high heels. I don't believe you did anything wrong. If a student is uncomfortable doing this pose have them perform an alternative against the wall.

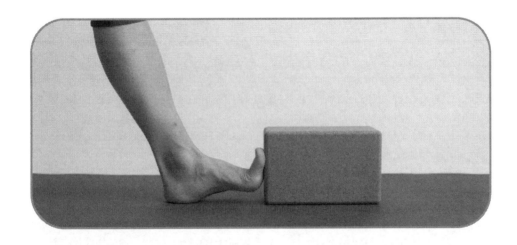

I told her my purpose was to gain flexibility in the toes for poses like lunge, and that it was still possible to engage the arch while in this position. However, I really truly have no idea of the correct answer to her question, that makes sense and I think that is a good reason. What is your opinion?

Some believe that fascia on the bottom of the feet is connected to the rest of the fascia in the body and stretching the arches of the feet will instead keep the tissue mobile. I would recommend balancing the "toe curled under pose" with the opposite "toes pointing back pose" while pressing the top of foot into the ground (to keep the front of the ankle engaged).

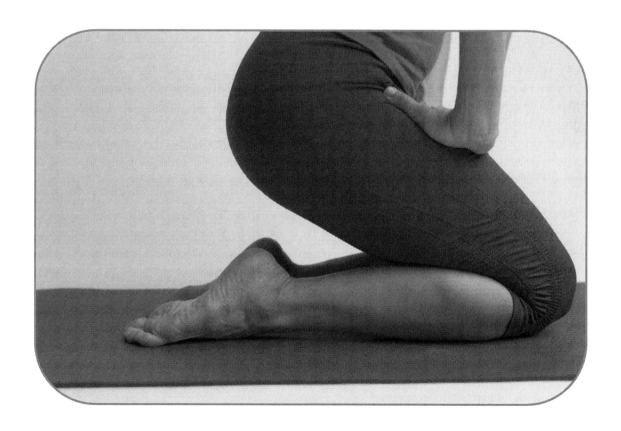

I think the idea of overstretching the arches and it being irreversible is a bit extreme. Flat arches (overstretched arches) tend to come from varied causes and generally develop with years of walking and standing with poor support, not overstretching the feet. My opinion about the physical therapist is that I understand where she is coming from. Physical therapists, including myself, are a bit guarded when viewing an extreme pose or exercise in a class setting. Since we work with an injured population, we start to think about our *one* patient who overstretched their arches, and we get nervous that everyone will.

We also work with patients individually, so we tend to get nervous when a group of people are given a position that appears extreme because we wonder if it is beneficial for every student. You should have listened to the "physical therapist voice" in my head when I first started taking yoga classes. Now that I have been a yoga teacher since 2010 my "physical therapist voice" has become less critical and more curious. I think you did a great job answering the question. It sounds like you explained why you do the pose to the degree that you understood it - which is perfect.

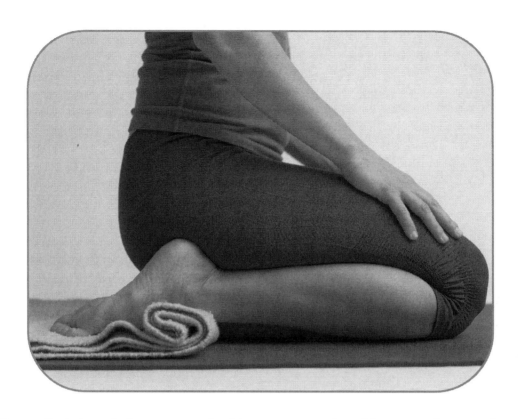

If you find that sitting on your heel is very uncomfortable across the top of your feet, try placing a small roll underneath your ankle.

I have weak ankles. Which yoga poses should I concentrate on or avoid?

When someone tells me they have weak ankles, I assume they have sprained their ankles. Ankles are commonly sprained by rolling on the outside of the ankle; this is called an inversion sprain. This sprain causes the deltoid ligament on the outside of the ankle to be overstretched. Repeated sprains can lead to a chronically overstretched ligament. The ankle joints are primarily stabilized by ligaments, especially the inside and outside of the ankle. Eversion sprains (rolling the inside of the ankle towards the ground) are less common secondary to the bony structures in the ankle and foot.

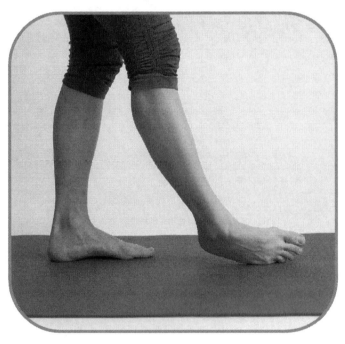

When an inversion ankle sprain occurs, the foot is plantarflexed (pointed) and inverted (pointed inwards), causing overstretching on the outer front area of the foot and ankle.

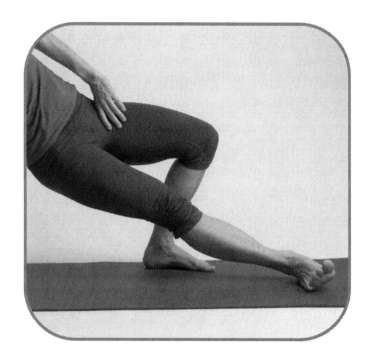

Yoga poses that can help strengthen the ankle are standing balance poses, emphasizing keeping the big toe mound down and inner heel rooted. Standing poses can be really helpful, especially if performed with the pinkie edge of your back foot against the wall. I recommend pressing the pinkie edge of your foot against the wall and even trying to pull the pinkie edge of your foot up the wall. This engages the peroneus muscles which stabilize the outside of the ankle.

As your ankle feels more stable, you can work with side plank and pigeon by pressing the pinkie of your bottom foot into the ground.

I would recommend avoiding lotus pose and being cautious with *virasana*. Make sure the pinkie edges of your feet are parallel to the long edge of your mat. In addition to strengthening your ankles, I would also recommend performing the foot opening exercises from pages 6-10 and working with keeping your hip muscles strong, specifically the *gluteus medius* (see page 27).

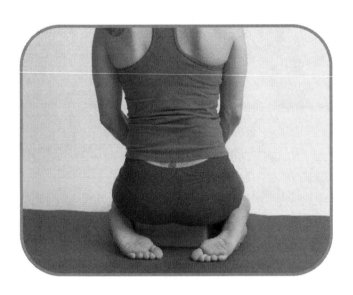

- Avoid relaxing your feet in *virasana*
- This is common when the top of the foot and ankle are tight
- Consider placing a small blanket roll underneath the front of the ankle and foot

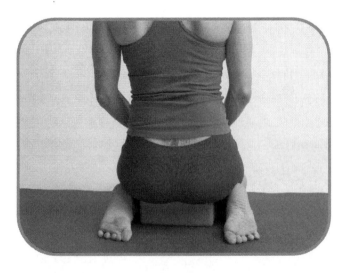

- Start with your feet pointing straight back, pinkie edges parallel with the long edges of your mat
- Watch your feet as you sit back
- Engage the outside of your shins by pulling your pinkie toes away from your hips

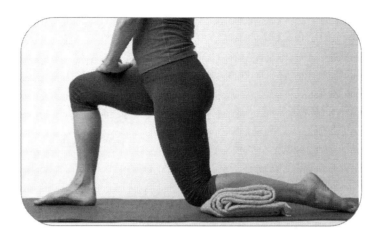

Instead of kneeling on your knee cap, place your shin on the blanket so your knee cap is floating above the ground. This can only be done if the foot is pointed.

Give yourself more time to recover, even twice as long. For example, if you exercise six days a week and only take one day off, try taking two days off. See if you feel better, stronger, or more well-rested.

What do teachers mean when they say "Root the inner edge of your foot"?

As stated above, it is quite common for students to sprain and therefore have weakness on the outside of their ankles. When yoga teachers ask students to root the inner edge of their foot, they are asking students to keep the big toe mound and inner heel steady to avoid the tendency to roll the ankles. When a student has high arches or supinated feet there is a tendency for them to roll their ankles outward and the cue to root the inner edge of their foot is very important. However, students who have collapsed, flattened, or pronated arch/feet will have a tendency to root the inner edge of their feet too much. These individuals would benefit from being asked to lift their arch and root the outer edge of their feet.

Students with supinated feet may find it more difficult to root their big toe mound and inner heel, while students with pronated feet may find it more difficult to root their pinkie toe mound and outer heel. I find it really important to acknowledge that not all cues are universal. It is important for yoga teachers to understand why the cues are used and make sure modification to the cues can be made to accommodate for each student in a yoga class. As a yoga student, it is similarly important to understand which cues apply to you and your practice.

I prefer cueing student on establishing a solid foot foundation. This allows students who have supinated or pronated feet to feel all 4 areas of the foot that should be equally rooted.

Establish good foot foundation.
Lift your heel and come onto the ball of your foot.
Root each point down in this order. Do this one foot at time.

1. Big toe mound
2. Outer heel
3. Inner heel
4. Pinkie toe mound

When I am doing a hamstrings stretch, I feel the stretch behind my knee. Is that normal?

I have heard this question from quite a few students. I can see the confusion, since hamstring stretches target the back of your leg and would include the back of the knee. The hamstrings and gastrocnemius attach to the medial (inside) and the lateral (outside) sides of the femur (upper thigh bone), and to the tibia (lower leg bone). There is a muscle at the back of the knee called the popliteus which helps to bend (unlock) the knee joint. The sciatic nerve also passes through the back of the knee. When my students ask me the above question I have them plantarflex (point their foot). If the pulling is relieved it is likely the sciatic nerve being that is being stretched.

The sciatic nerve is a long and large nerve running from the spine all the way to the heel of the foot. When students perform the hamstring stretch they are stretching the nerve in addition to stretching the hamstrings, glutes, and gastrocnemius. Nerves don't like to be stretched like muscles. When a nerve gets held in a stretched position it can get irritated. Nerves respond better to being flossed as opposed to stretched. Nerve flossing is alternating between a stretched position and a released position. Optimal nerve flossing treatment is the action between where you just start to feel a pull and feel the release of the pulling. I have my students alternate between plantarflexing (pointing) and dorsiflexing (flexing) the foot while keeping the hip and knee steady in their position.

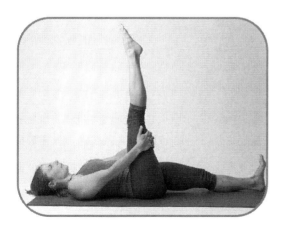
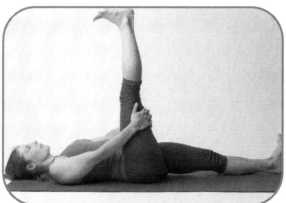

Another option is to keep the ankle and hip steady as you are flexing (bending) and extending (straightening) the knee. I tend to use the cue "soften the knee" vs. "bend the knee" to assure a small movement that will help find the optimal release position. Usually after a few repetitions of pointing and flexing the foot, the pull behind the knee resolves and the stretch is felt in the back of the thigh (hamstrings) or calf (gastrocnemius). To avoid irritating the sciatic nerve, it is best to continue to do nerve flossing when you feel the stretch behind the knee until you start to feel the stretch in the hamstrings (back of the thigh) or gastrocnemius (back of the lower leg).

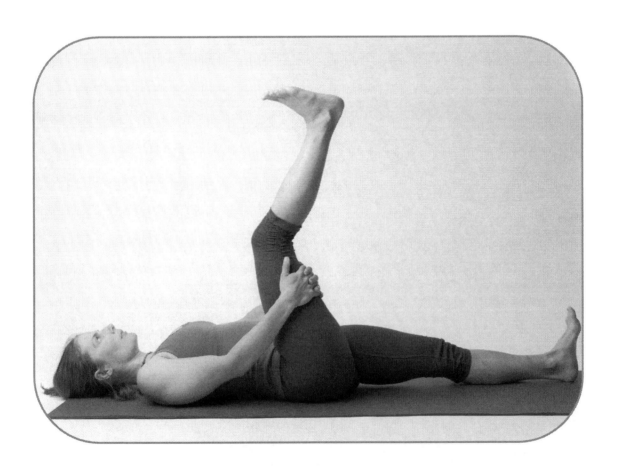

Can yoga help knocked knees?

Yes, I believe it can. Let's first define knocked knees, also called *genu valgus*. Knocked knees are common in children. This often resolves itself as the child ages. The angle of the femoral neck is called the Q angle and can affect the alignment of the femur. Women's Q angles are larger than men's due to women's pelvises being wider than men. Although a Google search about knocked knees is mostly associated with children, I often see knocked knees in adults. A big complaint I hear is "my thighs rub together because I have big thighs." I often find most students and clients with this complaint have a knocked kneed position. I define a knocked kneed position as the knees being narrower than the ankle. Flattened arches or pronated feet, weakness in the *gluteus medius*, and hyperextension of knees are the most common influences.

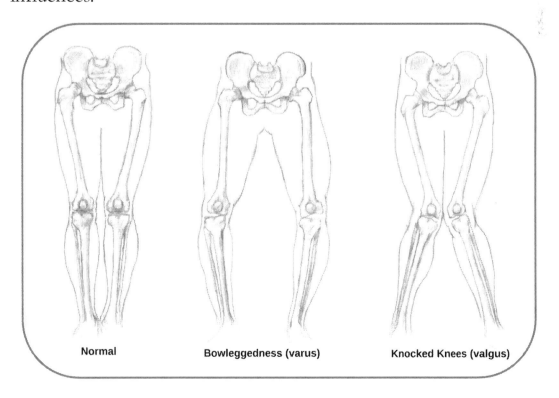

Mountain pose (*tadasana*), which is one of the first poses taught in yoga, is an excellent place to start. I have my clients first connect to their feet, bringing awareness to their feet pointing straight ahead, working to spread their toes and place more weight on the little toe edges of their feet while keeping their big toes down. Establishing a steady foundation in the feet is very important. I may even give my clients toe scrunching exercises with a towel, or have them lift the heel and bring the heel and big toe closer together in order to shorten the foot. Once I feel they have an understanding of their feet and a new awareness with what their feet are doing, we move up the leg toward the hip. The *gluteus medius* muscle is a hip abductor (bring the femurs away from each other) and it also internally rotates the femur (turn knee caps inward). I find most of my clients who have knocked knees have their feet wide with external rotation in their feet and femurs along with adducted knees (knocked knees).

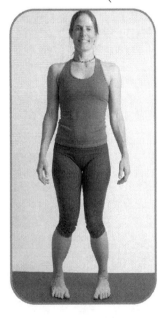
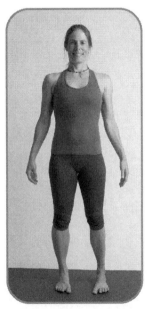

While standing, establish a solid foot foundation and make sure the feet are directly underneath the knees. Then I have them isometrically (act as though they are moving their heels but they are stuck on the sticky mat) pull their heels apart. This will internally rotate their femurs. I then have them pull their knees apart (abduction) as they still pull their heels apart. I often need to instruct my clients not to hyper-extend their knees, especially with internal rotation of the femurs. To help my clients understand abduction, I will often use a belt around the thighs, just above the knees, to give feedback that the thighs are pressing out. Mountain pose is just the beginning.

There are numerous yoga poses that can help strengthen the *gluteus medius* including single leg balances, like tree or baby dancer, along with the back leg in standing poses such as warrior 2, side angle, and half moon.

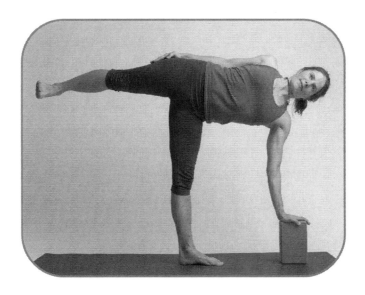

One of my students states she has a Baker's cyst. How will this influence her yoga practice?

The cause of a Baker's cyst is usually friction that creates deposit or fluids and tissue behind the knee joint. It can be quite alarming to find because it presents as a small to quite large lump behind your knee. The lump tends to be pain free but can occasionally be tender to the touch. The most annoying part of Baker's cysts is that they limit a student's ability to bend their knee fully. This will limit poses like child's pose, *virasana*, and twisted monkey. These students will likely need to use a strap to loop around their foot for any poses that ask them grab their foot with their hand. Having students place blankets underneath their hips in child's pose may help decrease pressure on the knee and effort in the pose. The size of the Baker's cyst can fluctuate and be present on in either knee or both. This change in mobility can frustrate to students who used to be able to grab their foot in certain yoga poses. This can be an excellent opportunity to share about the *niyamas* and *yamas* which are foundational to any yoga practice. Sharing the more subtle and deeper aspects of yoga may help the student become more accepting of their situation and body.

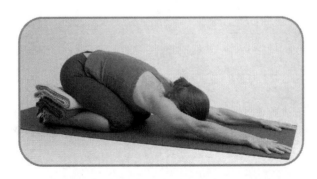

There is an instructor who believes we should not do any poses with straight legs, such as forward folds. She talks about it creating injuries, as our bodies are not meant to be in these positions. As a physical therapist, do you agree with this?

Great question and as is often the case, my answer would be "It depends." I find that more of my students, especially those new to yoga and who sit for a living, would benefit from bending their knees in forward folds.

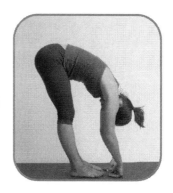

The reason a student would want to bend their knees in forward folds is to decrease the pull on the low back caused by tight hamstrings. The hamstrings are attached to *ischial tuberosities* (the sitting bones) which are at the bottom of the pelvis. When someone bends forward in a forward fold and their hamstrings are tight, the low back will round. Hence the hamstrings are pulling on the sitting bones, which pull the pelvis underneath (posterior tilt). A posterior tilt in the pelvis results in increased flexion (convexity) in the lumbar spine. This increased flexion in the lumbar spine can increase the risk for herniated discs in the lumbar spine and can contribute to increased low back and sacral iliac (SI) pain.

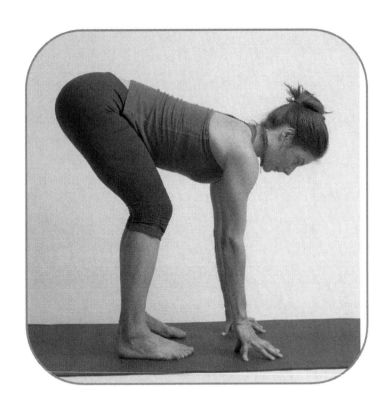

The benefits to bending the knees in forward folds are that it allows you to move and stabilize your pelvis, strengthen your back muscles, and help isolate the stretch to your hamstrings instead of your low back. In most cases of students with tight hamstrings, their low backs are overstretched and weak and their hamstrings are tight and functional, often stronger than the low back muscles. So by bending the knees, you are allowing the hamstrings to shorten and therefore not pull the pelvis into a posterior tilt. This allows the pelvis to tilt forward (anteriorly) and bring a more normal concave (extended) curve in the low back while you start to straighten your legs only to the degree that you can keep a curve in the low back and pelvis tilted forward. I apply this same awareness to down dog, which is considered a forward fold.

I also recommend the above steps to students who have really open hamstrings to ensure they are engaging their hamstrings as they perform their forward fold. I do believe bending your knees can be beneficial for new students, and even advanced students, to better articulate their poses and keep them safe. However, I hesitate to say "should not" or "never" since each person's practice is individual and unique. I believe a student should start with bent knees to bring awareness to their hamstrings before straightening their knees regardless of their level of flexibility.

If I strengthen my hip flexors, will that help loosen my hamstrings?

The hamstrings cross the hip joint (but are attached to the pelvis) and the knee joint. When the muscles are shortened this causes hip extension (back leg in lunge) or posterior tilt of the pelvis (often times performed when asked to tuck in your tailbone) and knee flexion. Some of the hip flexors (there are 9 of them) perform the opposite actions of the hamstrings which include, knee extension, anterior tilt of the pelvis (sticking your butt back behind you), and hip flexion (front leg in lunge). When a student performs forward fold pose with straight knees and bows forward, this stretches the hamstring over both the hip and knee joint and the low back. However, when one bends their knees and bows forward this stretches more of the glutes and to a lesser degree the low back and hamstrings.

When the hamstrings concentrically contract, the knee is flexed.

To isolate the hamstring specifically, a student would tilt their pelvis forward (contracting their hip flexors), sticking

> *Concentric is a shortening muscle contraction—origin and insertion move towards each other. In the case of the hamstrings, the* ischial tuberosities *(pelvis) move towards the tibia (lower leg).*

their butt back behind them, while keeping this tilting of the pelvis and straightening their knees only to the degree that they keep their pelvis tipping forward (hip flexor engagement).

The hip flexors flex the hip (knee to chest), bring your torso forward towards your thighs, and tilt the pelvis forward. It is important to be aware of what is happening in the pelvis and low back. Your low back and pelvis should stay steady and slightly tilted forward creating a concave (extended) curve in the low back while performing hamstring stretches. This action of stability is enforced by the hip flexors and back extensors. Strengthening the hip flexors and back extensors also helps with reciprocal inhibition which is a neuromuscular technique in which engaging the opposite muscle group (in this case the hip flexors and back extensors) will release the contraction of the hamstrings. This technique is used during triangle pose when students are asked to lift their knee cap or engage their quadriceps while stretching this hamstring in triangle pose. Therefore, strengthening your hip flexors has the potential to improving your hamstring mobility and protecting and even strengthening your low back.

For a video on stretching your hamstrings using your hip flexors, visit

http://www.yogaistherapy.com/stretching-hamstring-using-hip-flexors/

Yoga Therapy Tip

Incorporate hip mobility into your daily life. Work to move your hip in all its possible directions. Hip mobility is important to maintain healthy blood supply, smooth joint surfaces, and keep hip musculature from getting bound up and tight. These can also be performed standing.

In sitting,

- Bring your knees together and walk your feet apart (internal rotation),

- Bring your ankle over your opposite knees and let your knee move out (external rotation)

- Hug your knee towards your chest (hip flexion)

- Sit on the side edge of a chair and stretch foot behind you (hip extension)

- Bring your knee together or even cross your ankles (adduction)

- Bring your legs far apart (abduction)

Every time I try to bend my knee and grab my foot behind me, I get a cramp in the back of my leg. So in yoga class any time we are doing a standing thigh stretch or baby dancer pose, I just bend my knee without grabbing my foot. What can I do to avoid this cramping in the back of my thigh?

I am sorry to hear about your thigh cramping every time you try to perform baby dancer or a standing thigh stretch. It sounds as though either your hamstring (back of your thigh above your knee) or your *gastrocnemius* (calf muscle) is cramping. The hamstring muscles take the thigh into extension (move the knee back from the hip) and knee flexion (bend knee). When a muscle is shortened quickly it will likely cramp. Cramping is more common when the muscle we are asking to shorten is already tight.

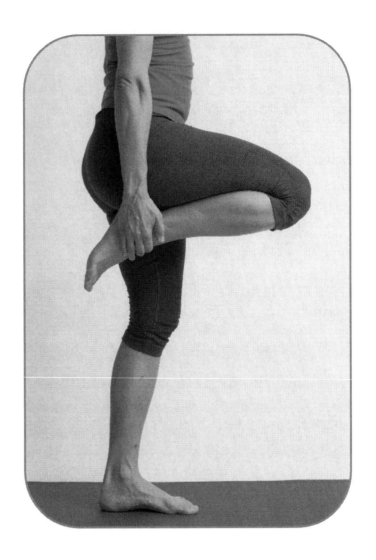

One way to avoid cramping the hamstring is to only perform one action at a time. So instead, lift your knee in front of you, bend your knee, bringing your heel towards your hip and then point your knee towards the ground. When the knee is brought forward, the hip is flexed (which is the opposite of extending) and the hamstrings are in a lengthened position. This allows one to bend the knee without cramping the back of the thigh. If this modification continues to cause cramping in the back of the leg then it is likely the calf that is cramping.

The *gastrocnemius* (calf muscle), like the hamstring, crosses two joints (the knee and the ankle) and flex the knee and plantarflexes the ankle (pointing the foot). To avoid cramping the calf, keep the toes pulling towards the shin (dorsiflexion) as the knee bends. Keep in mind that getting into and releasing out of poses are when most students are injured during their yoga practice. Therefore, it is important to be mindful of the body and any discomfort that may occur when entering and exiting a pose. It is ok to enter a pose in a different way than the teacher instructs as long as it is safe.

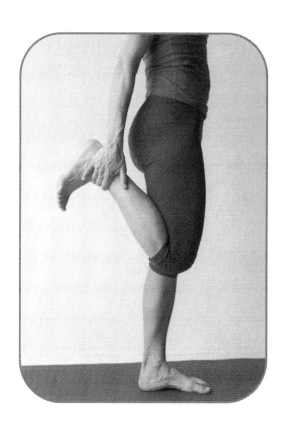

I feel a popping on the outside of my hip and I swear it is my ball and socket. It happens when I stand up from a sitting position. I didn't injure my hip, and I don't where it came from. What do you think is happening?

I have received this question quite often from students and clients of all ages. The hips have many muscles and tendons crossing across a ball and socket joint. Usually when the ball and socket of the hip is affected, the student will have pain deep inside their groin (bikini line) and will also have limitations in joint mobility. Here's a list of areas of the hip and likely causes of pain:

> **Anterior (front):** Hip flexors strain or tightness, labrum tear
>
> **Posterior (back):** Hamstring pull, sciatica, piriformis syndrome
>
> **Lateral (outer):** Iliotibial (IT) band tightness, *gluteus medius/minimus* or *tensor fascia lata* strain
>
> **Medial (inner):** Adductor strain

This is a very general list of areas that may be affected. A student can also have pain that radiates into the hip which is coming from the low back or a pelvic imbalance. The fact that you hear something "popping" on the outside of your hip is likely your tight IT band "popping" over your greater trochanter (boney prominence). The pain is likely from the bursa (fluid filled sac which helps tendons move over boney prominences) being irritated. I have some students who were concerned that their hip was dislocating, which I imagine is how it may feel.

The hip is a very stable joint surrounded by layers of muscles and held together by strong ligaments. I have only seen hips dislocate following a total hip replacement, a traumatic accident, or if a student has a connective tissue disorder.

I have pain along the outside of my hip. Should I have an x-ray to see if I have arthritis?

Pain on the outside (lateral) side of the hip is likely NOT from hip arthritis; rather, it is likely due to hip bursitis. When a person has significant hip arthritis the pain is felt deep inside the groin area, and they tend to present with decreased flexion (bending forward at the waist), rotation (knee pointing in while foot is out, knee pointing out while foot is in), and abduction (movement out to the side) of the hip joint. This specific limitation in range of motion of the hip is referred to as a capsular pattern. Capsular patterns can be indicative of hip arthritis. Hip bursitis is the result of the Iliotibial band (IT band) being tight, causing irritation of the bursa. This pain is often relieved by rest, postural correction (turning feet & knees straight ahead when sitting, standing, or walking), and self-massage and stretching to the IT band.

I would recommend obtaining a foam roller, preferably 5-6 inches in diameter, which can be purchased at any sporting goods store. My recommendation is to start slow, and laying the outside of your thigh on the roller, move forward and back then eventually up and down. When moving up stay below the hip crease, to avoid irritating the bursa and when going down, stay just above the knee. This is very uncomfortable if you have never done this before so take it easy. I often find students are more compliant if they have a soft roller instead of a hard roller. A soft roller can be purchased at OPTP.com.

Regarding where this tightness of the IT band came from: it is quite common in both active and inactive individuals. People who run, bike, or hike, or those who sit for long periods of time with knees splayed out likely have tight IT bands. Those who stand with their toes pointing out can also develop this.

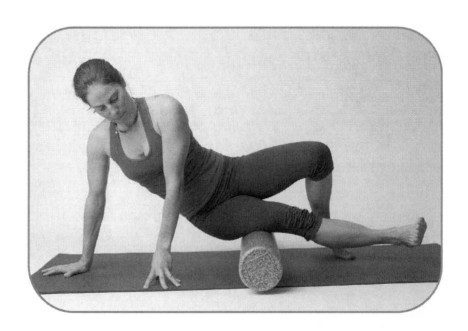

The IT band is a large piece of fascia which originates from a small muscle belly called the *tensor fascia latae* (TFL). It attaches to the fibula (outer shin) just below the knee. Since the *tensor fascia latae* has a very long tendon (the IT band), it can be tricky to stretch. One of the best techniques is to do self-massage with a roller. To see if your IT bands are tight, take your fingers to the outside of your thighs and notice if it feels soft, hard or stiff. Then dig your fingers in a little more and see if it is tender. Run your fingers up and down your outer thighs (stay away from hip crease and stay above the knee joint). The IT band and TFL can limit forward folds, hamstring stretches, external rotation in poses like pigeon, internal rotation in poses like cow face pose, and create challenges in keeping your knees hugging into the midline with backbends and quadriceps stretches. Addressing IT band tightness can not only relieve pain, it can improve your asana practice.

Receive one to two bodywork treatments per month. Massage and Myofascial release are excellent compliments to your yoga practice.

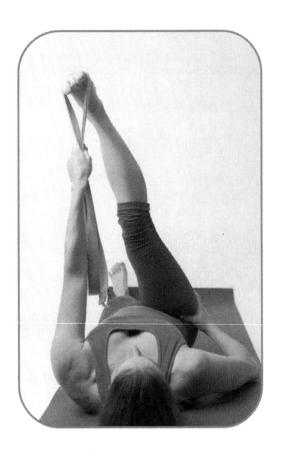 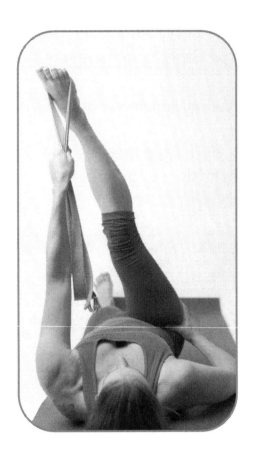

I find one of the best ways to stretch the tissues connected to the IT band is to come into a supine hamstring stretch (*supta padangusta*) and place both straps into the opposite hand. Then pull the right foot aligned with the left shoulder and pull your right foot towards your left shoulder while you push your right hip towards the end of your yoga mat with your right hand. This stretch is often felt along the outer shin, behind the knee, and along the outer thigh. There may be some burning discomfort with this stretch, and I would recommend pointing your foot, alternating pointing and flexing your foot, or backing away from the pose.

My partner is taking a yoga teacher training course. They are doing one weekend a month for about six months. She is on the second month, and she had a baby fourth months ago. She is having some problems with her hips and knees being sore. She thinks that maybe doing lots of yoga right after having a baby stretched her tendons out when she still had hormones that made her extra stretchy. What are your thoughts?

Ligaments and tendons become more elastic from hormones secreted while a women is pregnant and this continues even after she has given birth, especially if she is breastfeeding. This increased elasticity may appear to be an advantage to practicing yoga since it allows a person to go further in their poses. However, overstretching or hanging on the ligaments and tendons is common and is likely causing her discomfort. Knees tend to be the most common area for this since the knee has numerous ligaments and bursa. The outer hip is another common area to feel pain because of the Iliotibial band (IT band) which is a very long tendon running from the hip to the outer knee. The muscle belly of the IT band, the *tensor fascia latae,* originates from the pelvis. As a woman's pelvis expands and changes for child birth, this shifts the angle at which the tendon is attaching and can cause an increased pressure on the bursa. A bursa is a fluid-filled sac located between ligaments/tendons and boney areas. The bursa's purpose is to help ligaments and tendons glide and move smoothly over boney areas.

However, if the bursa is overly pressured it causes irritation and decreased movement. It becomes inflamed and causes pain. To avoid discomfort or overstretching of ligaments and tendons, I would recommend having your partner activate her feet more, especially with hip opening when the knee is out to the side, like pigeon pose or thread the needle. I would also recommend bringing more awareness of hyperextension in her knees with straight leg poses like *supta padangustasana*, triangle, or tree. I would also advise her to think more about keeping the muscles engaged while stretching as opposed to stretching as much as she can.

I am pregnant with my second child and about halfway through my pregnancy I started to get sciatic nerve pain down my right leg and I can barely put weight on my leg. Is there anything I can do about it?

Congratulations on your pregnancy! As a woman's pregnancy progresses, her body begins to change and prepare for birth. The area where the pelvis and sacrum join is called the sacroiliac joint (SI joint). This area starts to move and shift as a woman's pregnancy progresses due to hormone changes and increased weight to the front of pelvis. There is a muscle called the piriformis that is attached to the underside of the sacrum. The piriformis has a close relationship with the sciatic nerve. It is thought to protect the sciatic nerve and also helps with external rotation and abduction of the hip joint while standing or sitting in a chair. When the pelvis changes, the orientation and pull of the piriformis increases. This can cause tightness or strain on the piriformis muscles, which may increase pressure on the sciatic nerve. I would recommend first to bring awareness to how you are sitting or standing and try your best to keep your knees and toes pointed straight ahead.

I recognize this can be especially difficult in sitting. However, do your best to keep your knees from falling open even if you have to widen your knees to do so. I would recommend stretching your piriformis muscles in a seated position by crossing your ankle on top of your opposite knee, then try to keep an engagement in your hip muscles by placing your same hand underneath your open knee, creating resistance between your hand and knee in order to engage your outer hip. Maintain this as you allow your knee to move towards the floor. Keep your toes pulling up towards your knee (flexing your foot) to protect your knee joint.

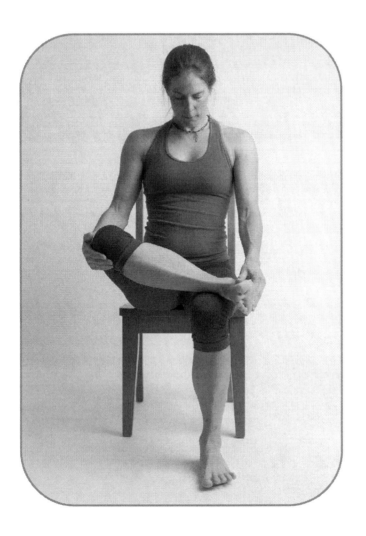

I would also recommend squeezing your gluteus muscles while you are shifting weight onto your symptomatic side and taking frequent standing breaks between long periods of sitting.

I have been told I have piriformis syndrome which is causing pain to shoot like sciatica down my leg. I was told to do pigeon pose but it makes the pain worse. If the piriformis is tight why would pigeon pose make it worse? What yoga poses can I do to help this?

Piriformis Syndrome is often misdiagnosed or referred to as sciatica. Sciatica is formally diagnosed by impingement occurring in the spine which can cause pain or numbness to radiate down one leg. Piriformis syndrome occurs when the piriformis muscle tightens and presses on the sciatic nerve causing pain and numbness down the leg.

Sciatica and piriformis syndrome have very similar symptoms and can be diagnosed by a physical therapist with few special tests. Once the student knows that they have piriformis syndrome there are some special consideration when doing yoga.

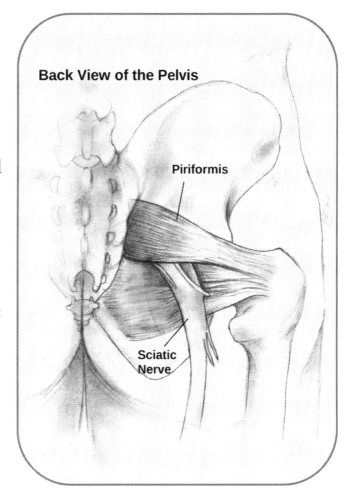

First, let's talk about the piriformis muscle. It is a deep hip muscle and has a very close relationship to the sciatic nerve. In fact, its job is to protect the sciatic nerve. When the piriformis is tight people often describe it as a deep pain in the center of their *gluteus* (butt cheek) or it feels like they are sitting on a ball on one side. The piriformis muscle originates on the front (underside) of the sacrum and attaches to the lateral (outer) aspect of the hip. There is a left and a right piriformis muscle and if one side becomes tighter than the other this can create pain in the SI joint (sacroiliac). Sometimes stretching the piriformis muscle helps the symptoms of the leg improve. In your case stretches make your symptoms worse, which tells us that your piriformis muscle may be overstretched.

> *While sitting, bring awareness to the levelness in your pelvis. Bring awareness to which sitting bone* (ischial tuberosity) *has more weight on it. Try to make the weight even between the right and left sitting bone, even if your legs are crossed.*

To investigate this further, rest on your back and cross your right ankle over your left knee (reclined pigeon). Keep your pelvis steady and maintain a neutral curve in your low back by keeping a slight arch away from the ground. Notice how far you are able to open your knee towards the right, and notice your pelvis again. There is a tendency to shift the pelvis when the knee opens to the side; the pelvis tends to move with the knee. Stop at the point where you can no longer keep your pelvis steady, then perform this pose on the left side. Compare and find the side that is tighter or causing symptoms (stop at the point just before your symptoms start). Do the pose on the side that is most limited first, which may not be your symptomatic side.

Sustain the pose for 10 deep breaths. You may feel a stretch along your outer butt cheek/hip. Then perform this pose on the other more flexible side only to the same degree as the tight side, like a mirror image. Place your hand on the outside of the knee and press your knee into your hand to engage the muscles without moving your knee any further out. Sustain this for 10 deep breaths. This technique can help bring balance to your piriformis muscles.

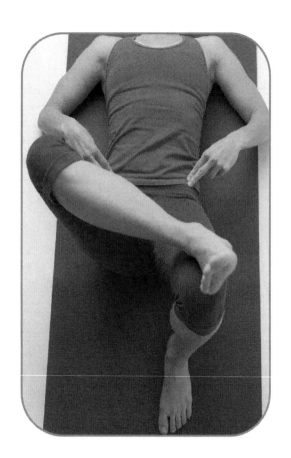
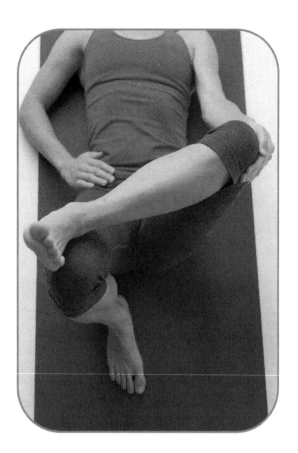

This technique can help bring balance to your piriformis muscles.

Another way to help bring stability and balance to the piriformis muscles is by strengthening the *gluteus medius*. When the *gluteus medius* muscles are strong, they stabilize the pelvis, especially when weight is shifting right and left. When these muscles are weak, the piriformis muscles try to compensate by contracting to stabilize the sacrum. The sacrum and pelvis (ilium) are attached by the SI joint. Since the *gluteus medius* is a larger muscle that originates from the pelvis, this compensation strategy can lead to the piriformis fulfilling a role it is not qualified to do. Since the piriformis' purpose is to protect the sciatic nerve when the muscle tightens up, it causes piriformis syndrome. You may consider concentrating on strengthening the *gluteus medius* and avoiding stretching the piriformis.

To bring more balance to your hip external rotators, place a looped strap around your big toes during savasana. *This simple trick can help prevent and treat piriformis syndrome.*

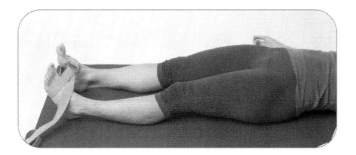

You have mentioned in your classes that there are three ways of bringing balance to the muscles in your body. What are the three ways and why?

I mention this frequently in class and I start by talking about how we are almost always trying to open our tighter side. What I propose is backing away from opening our flexible side, in order to allow our tighter side to catch up (or at the very least bring more balance to our body). I use these techniques most often with hip opening poses because I tend to hear the most complaints about the "bad" or tight hip. The three ways to bring balance are as follows:

1. Perform stretching twice as much the time or repetitions on the tight side while only once on the flexible side.

   - Although this may seem like it would lead to more imbalance, I have found this to help bring balance by allowing the tighter side more time to open.

2. Perform stretching on the tight side first then perform to the same degree on the flexible side. Engage to create a sensation and more stability on your open side.

   - This one is tricky and involves noticing when you first begin to feel a stretch to determine which side may be tighter. I find most of my students have a hard time figuring out which side is tighter because they move into the stretch too quickly.

3. Perform stretching on the tight side and perform a strengthening exercise on the flexible side. Stretch only the tight side, while strengthening only the flexible side.

   - This one is the most challenging for my students who like balance and keeping things "even Steven." This may be more of my physical therapy side coming out.

Regarding your tighter side, most students believe they have a "tight" hip. I have found usually both hips have tight areas. For example, someone may have tighter right hamstrings, which means the opposite muscles on the front of the body (the right hip flexors) would be more open. If their right hip flexor is more open, then left hip flexor may be tighter which creates more openness in their left hamstrings.

For a video on how to address muscle imbalances in your yoga practice, visit
http://www.yogaistherapy.com/3-ways-to-address-muscle-imbalances-in-your-yoga-practice/

I have attended your classes and notice you emphasized the "tight" side being a good thing and often recommended backing off on the looser side. Why?

I find most of us who attend yoga after a period of time find out we have a tighter hip, shoulder, or twist towards one side. This tighter side or action ends up being something we perceive as holding us back in our yoga practice. Yoga asana focuses on opening the joints and muscles, so when we are considerably restricted on a side we tend to label this side as the "bad" side. This can progress further toward being frustrated at that area of your body, and in a way, not giving it the credit it deserves.

This can become your guide in your yoga practice. A great way to redirect your frustration is to back off on the side that can do more. This will help "even out" both sides of the body. Simply producing the same degree of the pose on your looser side gives your body a chance to find equanimity. Friendly warning: your ego will likely want to boycott this opportunity since we often celebrate and honor the side that is more open because it gets us further in the pose.

I find the best poses to play with these techniques are one-sided hip stretches like pigeon and *supta padagustasana* (supine hamstrings stretch). I would recommend using a strap even if you can touch your foot. However, I would encourage you to practice these techniques in any yoga pose of your choice. As you

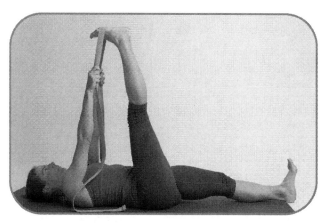

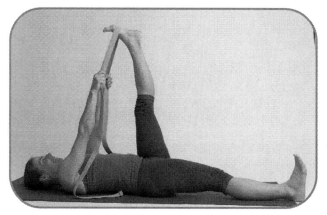

can see in the pictures, my right hamstrings allow me to go further into the pose. Therefore, I would back off the stretch on my right side which will bring more balance to my hamstrings and allow my left hamstrings to be equal to my right. I find taking pictures of myself or practicing where I can see myself in a mirror while doing the pose is helpful for me to see my imbalances.

Supta padagustasana means "knee-to-nose pose" and is one of the best stretches for low back pain

What are hip precautions after total hip surgery?

Depending on the surgery, there are three options: no hip precautions, posterior hip precautions, and anterior hip precautions. Each surgeon will have different time frames regarding how long their patients should follow hip precautions; I would recommend asking your student or client if their surgeon has approved the patient to resume normal activities. It is always a good idea to be aware of hip precautions even after the student/client is approved for normal activities.

No hip precautions means just that: no restrictions. However, I would still get approval from the surgeon before starting a yoga program.

Posterior Hip Precautions

* No bending past 90 degrees at the waist,
* No crossing your legs (even at the ankle),
* No internal rotation (turning your toes/knee cap inward).

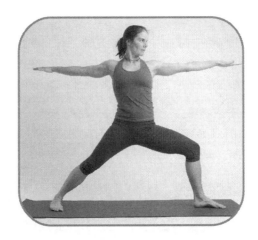

These precautions make sun salutations, forward folds and a variety of hip openers unsafe until one's restrictions are lifted. When a person returns to yoga after a total hip replacement with posterior hip precautions, I would recommend keeping their feet and knees wide in all forward folds, including child's pose, and instead only bending to ninety degrees at the hips. Half forward fold is a great starting place. I would be very cautious with hip openers like pigeon or any other poses which stretch the outer and posterior hip musculature. Safe poses include backbends such as bridge pose, and standing poses such as Warrior 2 and Tree pose. I would not recommend moving into triangle or side angle poses because the front hip is flexed beyond ninety degrees at the waist.

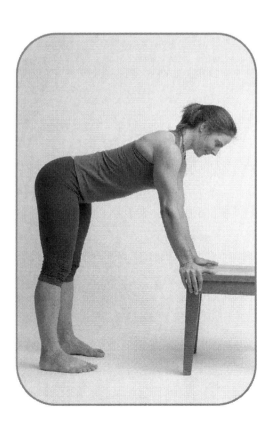

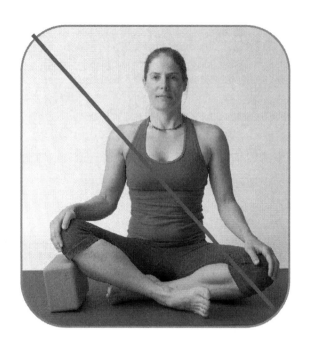 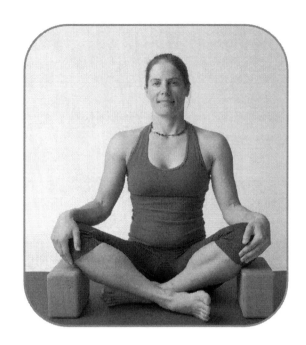

*When supporting your body, support both sides
even if it seems like only one side needs it.*

Anterior Hip Precautions

* No hip extension (reaching your leg behind you)

* No abduction (bringing your leg out to the side away from the body)

* No external rotation (turning toes and knee outward)

These precautions provide more freedom in daily activities. However, starting back to a yoga practice may be more challenging. With these students I would recommend avoiding backbends, stretching of the anterior thigh like *anjaneyasana* or even simple lunge pose, wide length poses (beyond hip distance width), and hip openers involving the knee moving away from the midline, like *badhakonasana*.

Badhakonasana, or cobbler's pose: the bottom of the feet are together while the knees are apart

---

This one sounds simple, but it takes practice:
When someone gives you something, whether it is a verbal gift or
a material gift, say thank you first before saying anything else.

When a person returns to yoga after a total hip replacement with anterior precautions, I would continue to use caution when introducing anterior hip stretches. Work first with keeping the knee directly underneath the hip then slowly work with moving the knee back from the hip. Safe poses would included forward folds, like child's pose, along with down dog and twists with knees together.

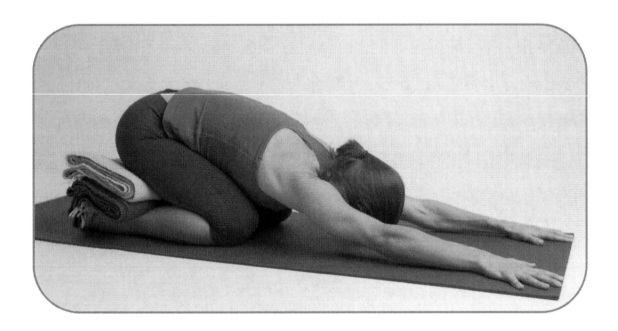

I have had a total hip replacement. I love to practice yoga. However, I really don't like balance poses. I know you would tell me to do them to acquire strength. Why, and what should I do?

In asana we try to avoid poses that we don't like or that we are not good at. I go to a public yoga class because if I am left at home to do my practice, I only practice what I am good at or what I like to do. Depending on how long ago your hip surgery was and what approach the surgeon used, your *gluteus medius* muscle may have been cut or stretched during surgery. The *gluteus medius* muscle stabilizes the pelvis when balancing on one leg and this tends to be weak in students who have had a total hip surgery with a posterior approach. This muscle can be strengthened by standing on one leg, which means standing balance poses are probably most challenging and may be the best way for you to strengthen a key hip muscle. Interestingly enough, there has been an association between *gluteus medius* weakness and piriformis syndrome.

One way to isolate the *gluteus medius* muscles is to perform leg lifts against the wall. Rest your body with your back along the wall, placing your weaker leg on top. You may bend your bottom leg for balance. Bring your top heel to the wall and keep your heel touching the wall the whole time as you lift and lower your leg slowly.

Keep your knee cap and toes pointing straight ahead with your foot flexed. Keep pressing your heel against the wall to engage the back of the thigh. This is safe to do following total hip surgery if you have posterior hip precautions.

If you have anterior or no hip precautions, you can progress by turning your toes and knee cap towards the ground (internal rotation) and slowly lift and lower. This should not be done if you still have posterior hip precautions. You should feel the muscles of your lateral (side) posterior (back) top hip.

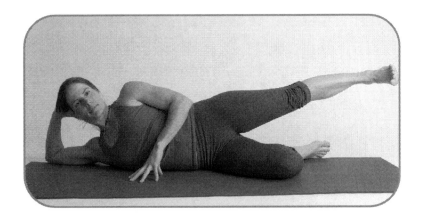

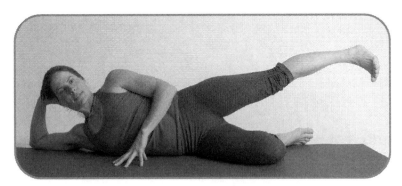

It is common for the hip flexor to want to help, and you may feel the anterior (front) muscles of your hip working. If this is the case, press your heel into the wall and imagine your lateral posterior muscles (side back butt check) of your top hip working. If this exercise is too challenging lying on your side against gravity, you can perform this pose on your back and slide your leg out to the side and back towards the center. Do not internally rotate if you have posterior hip precautions.

Another technique to strengthen your *glute medius* is standing with an isometric contraction. Isometric activation is an activation of the muscle with little or no movement seen. This is one of the three different activations that a muscle is able to perform. Isometric contraction is used for stabilizing and to create endurance. I like to call this posture "Stance." Start with your feet pointing straight ahead and isometrically (imagine your feet are glued to the ground) pull your heels apart. Then, keeping your heels pulling apart, pull your knees apart isometrically. There may be minimal movement observed like while you pull your heels away from each other your knees may point inward slightly (internal rotation of the hips) and then when you pull your knees apart (abduction of the hips) your knees will be pointing straight ahead.

Here are few pointers to assure you aren't overdoing it and compensating with other strong muscles:

- Keep your big toe mound rooted to the wall the whole time; there is a tendency to roll out on the ankles.

- Soften your knees; there is a tendency to lock the knees when pulling the heels away from each other.

- Draw your knees straight out to the side (hip abduction); there is a tendency for the knee caps to roll outward into hip external rotation. Be sure to keep the knee caps pointing straight ahead while drawing the knees out to the side.

- As you perform these actions, notice if you feel your lateral posterior hip area engaging. This is your *glute medius* muscles. This is a technique you can use while standing at work or doing the dishes.

Another way to access your *glute medius* is in tree pose. I would recommend doing tree pose in front of the mirror. Don't forget this is a balance pose, so feel free to stand close to the wall. I recommend the wall be behind students. If balance is a concern for you, stand with your back against the wall and shift your weight onto your right leg.

Notice if your right hip starts to move way out towards the right. This is common compensation for weakness in the *glute medius* and allows students to use the tightness of their outer hip to keep them balanced. Before placing your left foot for tree pose, try to pull your right hip underneath you more. Use your left hand to place your left foot into your right inner thigh. Keep pressing your right inner thigh into your left foot. I often hear yoga teachers say "press your foot into your inner thigh" but be sure to also "press your inner thigh into your foot." Be aware that this may be more challenging for your balance in the beginning. However, once you establish steadiness and strength in your *glute medius*, all of your single leg balance poses will improve along with your transition while standing on one leg.

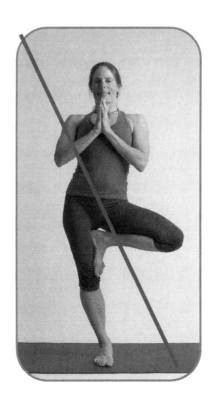 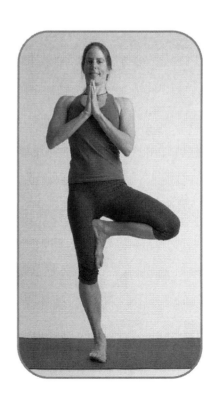

I am afraid to stretch after injuring my hamstrings and groin. This has been going on for several months. Do I stretch it or do I rest it? How do I know when to stretch a sore area of my body without causing further injury?

Hamstring pulls/injuries or groin injuries are a common injury among yoga students. After injury/overstretching/strain to your groin or hamstrings, most people note tenderness near the origin point of the muscle. The adductor muscles originate on the pubis bone and the hamstrings originate on the ischial tuberosity. The three hamstrings muscles come together to form a long tendon which is the common area of injury. The five adductor muscles do not have a common tendon and have a broader origin area which decreases the chances of injuring the whole muscle group. Both of these areas tend to cause deep-seated discomfort near the origin site when the muscle is stretched. For the adductors, this tends to be high up in the groin region usually near the bikini line area and for the hamstrings is just below the glute (butt cheek). After an overstretching or strain injury the body reminds us every time that we have an injury, especially when we stretch. As a result, we avoid stretching or activity completely and then the muscle further tightens and weakens.

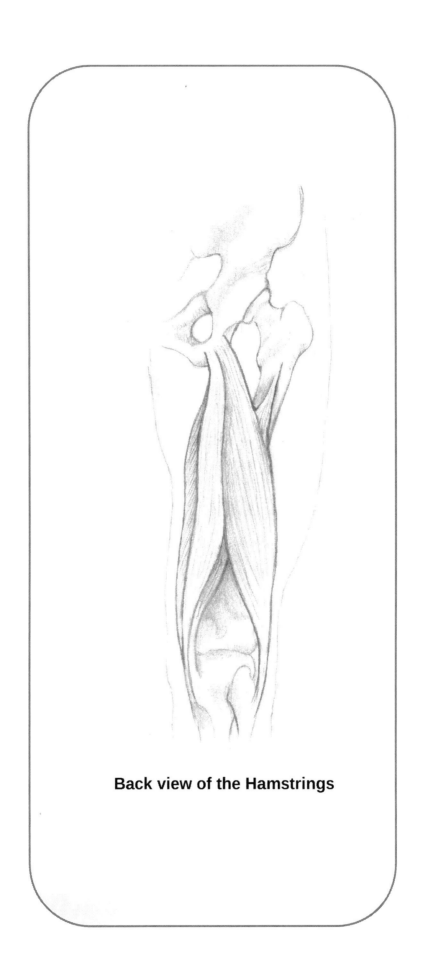

Back view of the Hamstrings

What I recommend to people following a hamstrings or adductor strain is to stretch with awareness. If you feel pain in the origin area as named above, then back off to avoid pain or further injury. The muscles need to be engaged while stretching to make any stretch following an injury safe. In standing forward fold, engage the hamstrings and draw your heel towards your hip (keep your knees slightly bent). In seated forward fold, press your heel down and isometrically (contraction with little or no movement) pull your heel towards your hip.

In standing poses or lunges, pull your heel back towards your back foot. When engaging the hamstrings, ensure you feel the muscle belly work. If you are unsure, place your hand on the middle part of your back thigh (muscle belly) and see if you feel the muscle engage.

You can approach the adductors in the same way. To engage the adductors, you will want to isometrically pull your feet or knees towards each other. Again, if you feel pain or discomfort in your upper inner thigh near the origin, back off and re-engage. Place your hand on your inner thigh between your knee and your groin and feel if the muscles are engaged. Then keeping this engagement, lessen the contraction enough to slowly start to stretch in the pose.

If at any point you feel a pain in the origin area, back off and re-engage the muscles and try again. In the beginning, you may not feel a stretch at all. Instead you may just feel your hamstring or adductor working. To prevent a muscle strain or to heal a muscle strain, the muscle must stay engaged to prevent overstretching and to re-establish strength and stability within the muscle belly.

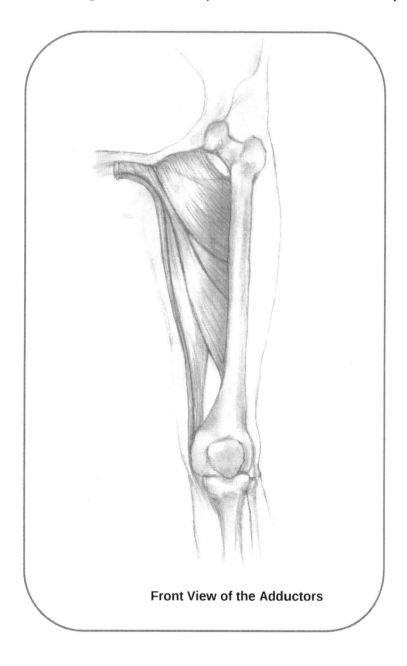

Front View of the Adductors

I have attended a few of your workshops and you are the only yoga teacher that I have met who recommends strengthening and stretching the hamstrings instead of only stretching tight hamstrings. How can I do this in my yoga poses?

I recommend strengthening and stretching all the muscles in the body. Just because a muscle is tight doesn't mean it is strong. I find most people are strong in a certain range of motion, and yoga poses give us an opportunity to create more strength in a larger range of motion. I oftentimes find the muscles on the front of the body including the quads and hip flexors are tighter and oftentimes stronger than muscles on the back of the body, including the glutes and hamstrings. This commonly occurs because a lot of activities are performed moving the body forward and therefore the muscles in the front of body are used more often than the muscles on the back of the body. I find this is often the case in yoga poses such as standing poses and backbends. One way to use your hamstrings more in yoga poses is to pull your front heel back towards your back foot in staggered foot poses. Your front heel will stay on the ground. Hopefully you will feel the back (underside) of your thigh engage. This creates a co-contraction of the quadriceps (top) and the hamstrings (underside) of the front thigh which will help you sustain the pose longer with more stability.

For a video on engaging your hamstrings in yoga poses, please visit

http://www.yogaistherapy.com/engagement-of-hamstrings-in-yoga-poses/

My hip flexors have recently become "grabby" in some seated and supine poses with knees bent (ardha matsyendrasana, supta balasana). *Surprisingly, they don't bother me in* navasana *or other ab work.) I also have been running a lot more lately. Do you think these two things are related? What can I do in terms of both my running form and yoga alignment to mellow out my hip flexors? I also don't want running to interfere with my yoga practice. What are your thoughts?*

Running and tight hip flexors are definitely related to each other, along with tightness in the glutes and hip rotators. When performing *navasana*, one combines the use of hip flexors and abdominals simultaneously. The basic position involves much less hip flexion than *ardha matsyendrasana* and *supta balasana* (double knees to chest). When hip flexors are tight they can feel "bunched" up when one fully flexes their hip (brings knee to chest). The cause of your grabby hip flexors can be from tight hip flexors, tight hip extensors (glutes/hamstrings), and tight hip rotators (piriformis/adductors). I would recommend running on flat surfaces and avoid running uphill so you don't use your hip flexors more than necessary. Another important question is what is your pelvis doing during these "grabby" times? The psoas and iliacus are primary hip flexors and are attached to the lumbar spine and pelvis. Therefore, the placement and stability of your pelvis in poses is very important.

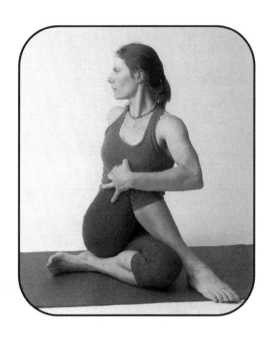 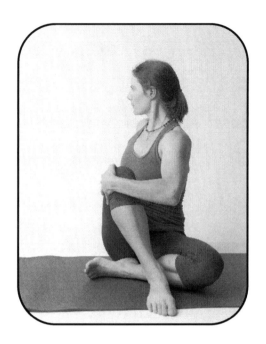

Rather than placing your front foot outside your opposite thigh in *ardha matsyendrasana*, bring your foot in front of your shin instead. Keeping this, hug both heels in toward your shin and opposite glute. Regarding your pelvic alignment, try playing with tilting your pelvis forward and back and see which relieves the grabby feeling in your hip flexor.

> *Bring awareness to the area of your body*
> *that maybe you are not so proud of and take time*
> *to brainstorm ways to improve your awareness to this area.*
> *For example, my glutes are my area.*
> *I am bringing more awareness to my glutes*
> *by squeezing my glutes while standing, walking, and sitting.*

In *supta balasana* (double knees to chest), I would recommend widening your knees and placing your hand behind your knees. With your hand underneath your knee pull your knee towards your chest and reach your hips towards the ground. Play with trying to create a curve in your low back (arch your low back away from the floor). I think running and yoga can be a great combination and complimentary to each other if they are performed correctly. It is key to assure you are stretching your hip musculature with awareness and stability in your pelvis.

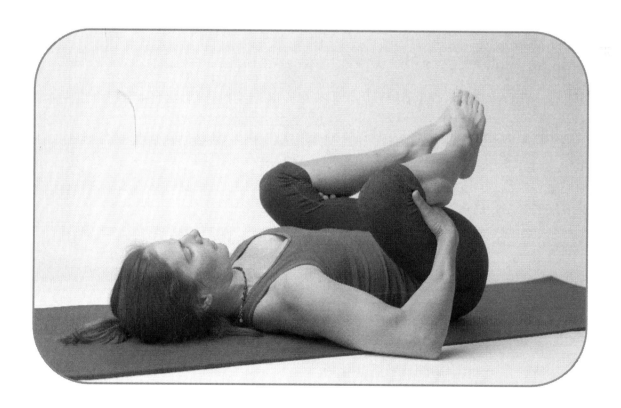

How do you avoid overusing your hip flexors in boat pose?

This is a common complaint when students perform boat pose. In addition to it just being a challenging pose, I choose not to teach boat pose in my back care classes because I find most of my students have tight hip flexors from sitting for a living. Unfortunately, boat pose contracts the already short and tight hip flexors which cause cramping and discomfort in the hip creases and could possibly lead to low back pain.

I am not saying students should never do boat pose and I feel boat pose has its place to connect students to their hip flexors. Most students will perform boat pose and complain of pain in the front of their hip crease or their low back. This is common because one of our major hip flexors, the psoas, originates on the lumbar (low back) vertebrae and when engaged can cause pain in the low back. In addition, the full form of boat pose is knees straight and toes as high as eyes. This position isolates the engagement of another hip flexor called the *rectus femoris* (which is one of the quadriceps muscles). When muscle shorten over both joints (hip and knee) that they cross the muscle will likely cramp unless accompanied by a co-contraction by the opposite muscles group. The hip flexors will work in boat pose. They have to, otherwise you couldn't lift your legs. Bending your knee or pressing your thighs into your hands to engage your hamstrings can help release the cramping in the front of the hips.

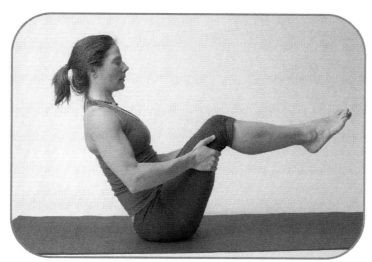

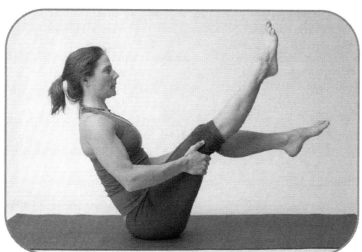

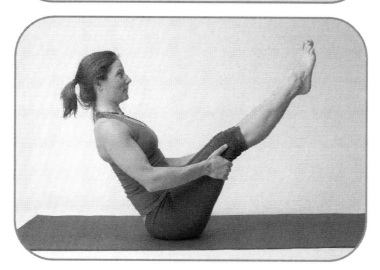

For techniques to help with boat pose, visit
http://www.yogaistherapy.com/boat-pose-technique/

two: *the upper body*

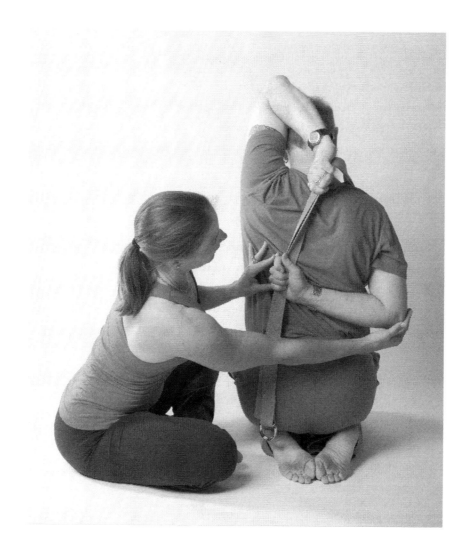

The upper body is asked to open and stabilize while doing yoga poses in a way that is foreign to normal everyday activities. This section will address questions about the shoulders, elbows, and wrist.

I notice when I am driving with my hands at 2 and 10 on the steering wheel my hands fall asleep. I have been tested for carpal tunnel and the tests are negative. The doctor said it may be thoracic outlet syndrome. Are there any yoga poses and breathing that I can do to help?

I am sorry to hear your hands fall asleep while you are driving… sounds like that could be dangerous. This can also happen when someone is practicing down dog or even just coming to hands and knees in cat and cow pose.

First, I recommend moving your hands into a more comfortable position, maybe the bottom of the steering wheel. If that doesn't cause your hands to fall asleep. I would also recommend using an armrest for each arm. Using armrests while driving, or even at your desk, can help support the weight of your arms to help relax your upper trapezius and neck muscles, and relieve tension. Thoracic outlet syndrome, which sounds scary, can be caused from your neck and shoulder muscles being tight which may cause your hands to fall asleep while your arms are held in one position for a period of time. I would recommend starting with a pectoralis release, diaphragm release, and practicing diaphragmatic breathing.

Diaphragmatic Breathing:
Inhale and allow your pelvis and belly expand.
Exhale and allow your pelvis and belly to recoil.

Pec release Place your opposite fingertips just outside your tank top strap into the tender area (under the armpit and in) *Inhale*: expand your breath into your upper chest *Exhale:* sink your fingers into the pec *Inhale:* release your fingers and expand your breath	Perform for 5-10 breaths on each side
Diaphragm release • Take the palm of your hands to the top of your ribs • Bring your finger just below the edge of your rib cage **Inhale**, allow the area under the ribcage to expand into your fingertips. • **Exhale**, curl your fingers underneath your ribs and grab the ribs. • **Inhale**, release your fingers. Allow the breath to expand and the area under the ribcage to expand. • Start with hands close to the middle and then move hands out to the side.	Perform for 3 breaths in each area, starting in the middle and move out to either side (2-3 areas)

To learn how to bring awareness to your diaphragm and pectoralis and perform diaphragmatic breathing, visit
http://www.yogaistherapy.com/release-for-your-neck-shoulders-and-diaphragm/

Why is yoga good for carpal tunnel syndrome?

I believe all of us have heard the statement "yoga can cure _____," (fill in the blank). Although I agree that a yoga practice can help improve a person's health, awareness, and pain, I think it is important to understand why. The carpal tunnel is located in the wrist between the carpal bones and reticulum (fascia).

The carpal tunnel has:

- 4 tendons of the *flexor digitorum profundus* (flexes fingers)
- 4 tendons of the *flexor digitorum superficialis* (flexes fingers)
- 1 tendon of *flexor carpi radialis* (flexes wrist and radial deviates)
- The median nerve (bring sensation and strength to the 4th & 5th finger)

Carpal tunnel syndrome is most commonly associated with people who type on the computer or people who use their hands and wrist in a flexed position. One of the benefits of yoga poses is that they take us out of our usual movement patterns. Since a fair amount of yoga poses are done with the hands on the ground with fingers spread and wrists in extension, yoga helps to stretch the tight flexors of the wrist and fingers. This is also why many students who first start yoga notice that their wrists are sore with weight bearing poses on their hands.

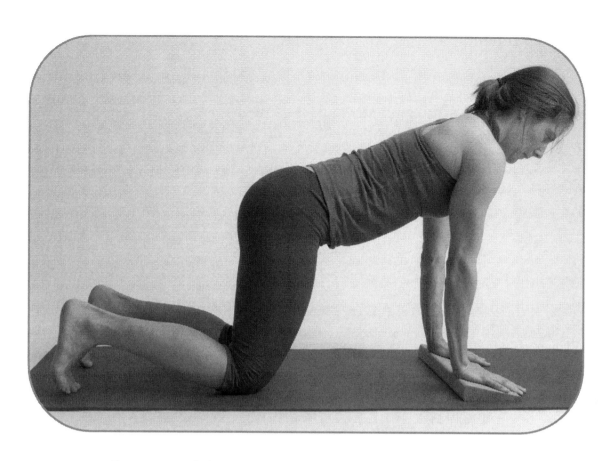

One way to help create more comfort in the wrist and hand is to elevate the palm of the hand on a blanket or wedge.

I find stretching the fingers individually into extension with the wrist also in extension, is a helpful way to address the 8 finger flexing tendons that run through the carpal tunnel.

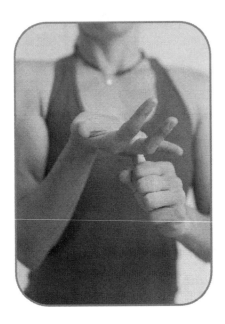 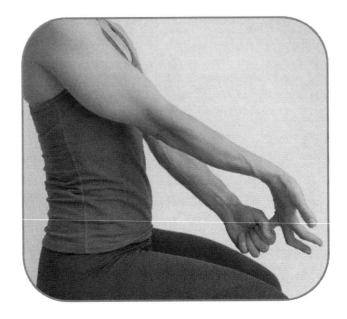

Start with wrist in extension, like you were a waiter holding a platter in front of you with your elbow bent. Take each finger one at time and pull the finger towards the ground while keeping your palm flat. You may feel a stretch all the way up your forearm which is where the muscle belly originates. You can also straighten the elbow to change the stretch. Sustain this stretch for one breath cycle (inhale/exhale) and then move to the next finger. You may be surprised how tight certain fingers are. I would recommend performing this stretch several times a day.

Can yoga help Tennis Elbow? What is Golfer's Elbow?

Yes, yoga can help with tennis elbow and golfer's elbow. Golfer's elbow is inflammation and overuse of the flexors of the wrist. It is called *medial epicondylitis* because the flexors of the wrist attach to the *medial epicondyle* of the humerus. Tennis elbow (*lateral epicondylitis*) is inflammation and overuse of the muscles that extend the wrist. One does not need to be a tennis player or golfer to have these conditions. They are quite common in construction workers and other professionals who use their hands to do their job. When someone has tennis elbow, it is recommend that they stretch their extensors by flexing the wrist and making a gentle fist with the hand. When the wrist is in extension this may aggravate symptoms of tennis elbow because it shortens the flexor of the wrist.

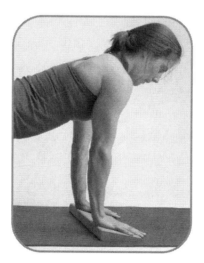

I would recommend that students use a wedge or a blanket underneath the palms of their hands to help decrease the wrist extension.

I would recommend for them to do stretches like placing the palms of their hands underneath their feet with elbows straight and with elbows bent (I would recommend taking any rings off).

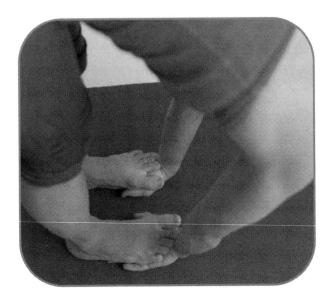

I would *not* recommend bearing full weight on wrists in a flexed position. Those with golfer's elbow likely benefit from hands and knees position with wrist extension because it would help stretch out the wrist flexors.

In addition to stretching the wrist flexors and extensors, I believe yoga helps tennis and golfer's elbow best by having students open their shoulder muscles, especially their pectoralis muscles.

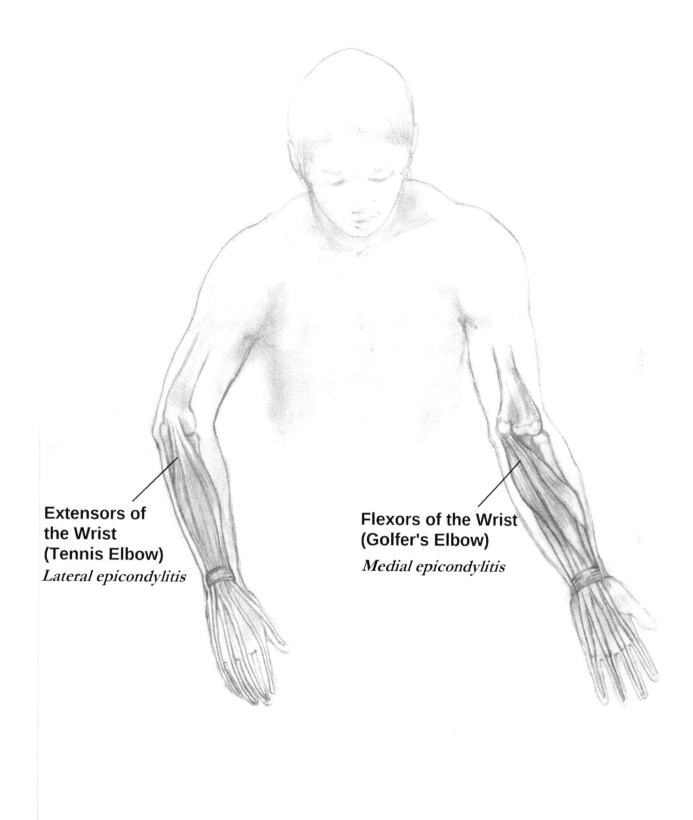

Neural tension release:
If you notice a pulling feeling during a stretch that feels like a string stretching or causes numbness, tingling, or burning sensation, try to soften your pose by softening your knee or elbow to release neural stretching.

You have talked about nerve flossing for the lower body, such as the sciatica nerve pulling the behind the knee in hamstrings stretches. Are there any nerve flossing techniques for the upper body?

Yes, there are nerve flossing techniques for the upper body that I find helpful for students who have pain or tingling in their arms and hands from carpal tunnel or thoracic outlet syndrome. There are nerves that originate in the neck and pass underneath the pectoralis minor muscle, and they split into 3 individual nerves. Since the nerves run underneath the pectoralis minor muscles when the pectoralis muscles (major/minor) are stretched, there may be numbness or tingling present during the stretch. I recommend releasing the pectoralis muscle by pinching or pressing on it (see page 133 for more details). The three nerves are the radial nerve, median nerve, and ulnar nerve. It is called nerve flossing instead of stretching because nerves don't liked to be pulled on, but instead, need to be glided through fascia and muscle tissue. When doing these techniques, be aware when coming into a pull or sensation and then release out of a pull or sensation, alternating between the sensation and no sensation. Sensation may include a subtle pulling of the tissue, tingling/numbness, or sometimes discomfort.

Radial Nerve Flossing

1. Pull your shoulder down away from your ear and straighten your elbow.
2. Bring your arm out to your side and behind you a bit and rotate your palm toward the ceiling (with arm rotating internally, biceps down towards the ground).
3. Pull your fingers up away from the ground towards your shoulder.
4. Side bend your head away from your arm.

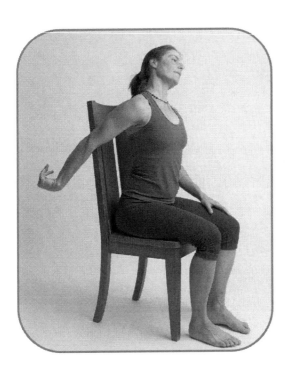
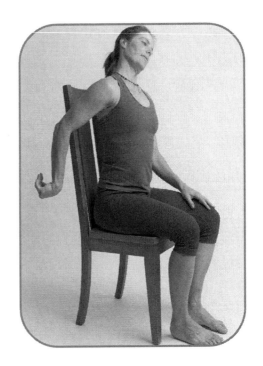

Releasing Radial Nerve Flossing

To release the pose, only move one joint at time. Keep the basic position. It is common to feel a stretching sensation in the forearm/elbow. Keep arm in steady position and do one of the following releases:

1. Release wrist from flexion
2. Bend the elbow
3. Shrug shoulder
4. Move head upright

- Notice which actions of the wrist, elbow, shoulder, or neck release any numbness, tingling, or pulling (that is felt). The release from the stretch should lessen the pull/stretch.
- Alternate between stretch and release for up to 1 minute.

Keep breathing and keep your face relaxed.

Median Nerve Flossing

1. Pull your shoulder down away from your ear and straighten your elbow.

2. Bring your arm out to the side and behind you and rotate your bicep up towards the ceiling (externally rotate).

3. Pull your fingers up towards the front of your forearm (extend your wrist).

4. Side bend your head away from your arm.

5. Notice if you feel any stretching feeling in your forearm.

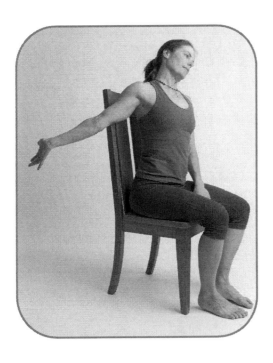
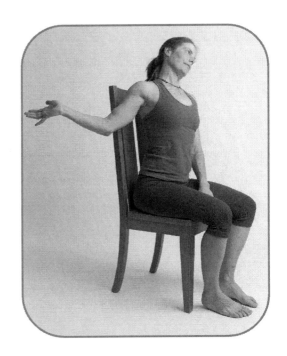

Releasing Median Nerve Flossing

To release the pose only move one joint at time, keep the basic position, and consider doing one of the following activities to release the position:

1. Release or flex the wrist.
2. Bend and straighten the elbow.
3. Shrug the shoulder.
4. Bring head upright and side bend.

- Notice which actions of the wrist, elbow, shoulder, or neck release any numbness, tingling, or pulling (that is felt). The release from the stretch should lessen the pull/stretch.
- Alternate between stretch and release for up to 1 minute.

> *Try a different yoga path. For example, try a meditation or pranayama class, or a class in a style of yoga you haven't tried or maybe even disliked in the past.*

Ulnar Nerve Flossing

1. Come into the position in the picture to the below on the left.
2. Pull shoulder down away from your ear. Notice where you feel a nervy-like stretch.

- If you feel this stretch in your neck, bring your head back to upright or shrug your shoulder.
- If you feel a stretch in your forearm or upper arm, release or straighten your elbow.
- Alternate between release and stretch.

Perform each of these techniques for up to one minute or for 10-12 breaths.

- Exhale, stretch. Inhale, release.
- It is common to have the arm feel tired after performing nerve flossing.

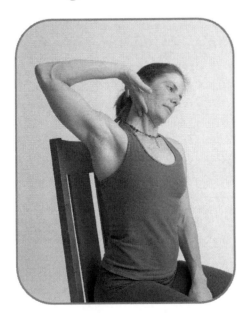
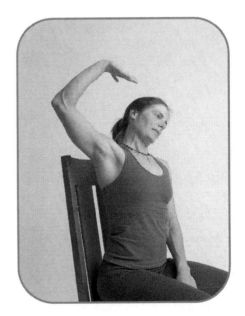

Stop if symptoms become more intense following this exercise.

What, really, does it mean to have "tight shoulders"?

Tightness in the shoulders can present itself in several different ways. Most people refer to tight shoulders in regards to functional mobility, reaching overhead, reaching behind to undo a bra, reaching in a back pocket, or poor posture. Usually tight shoulders are a result of tight pectoralis major and minor muscles since we tend to use these muscles to do most of our activities in life. Other reasons the shoulders may be tight are arthritic changes or injury involving the shoulder capsule. This condition is referred to as "frozen shoulder" and results in limited external rotation, abduction, and internal rotation of the shoulder. This usually affects only one shoulder and can be confused with having a tight shoulder. When the pectoralis muscles are tight it limits one's ability to reach arms overhead, interlace fingers behind the back, or perform backbends. Tight pectoralis muscles cause round shoulders and can lead to tightness and pain in the neck.

Bring awareness and balance to your shoulders. If you tend to carry a bag, purse, or objects with one hand, switch it up. If you have a backpack, use both straps.

Even though I am right-handed, I started brushing my teeth with my left hand, and notice it is starting to feel more normal

What is a shoulder impingement?

Impingement occurs when the *supraspinatus* muscle is pinched by the acromion process of the scapula. The most common symptom is pain on the outside of the shoulder with overhead movements, specifically when moving the arms out to the sides and overhead. Pain usually starts when the arm is at greater than ninety degrees of shoulder flexion or abduction. The shoulder joint is made up of four joints. The glenohumeral joint (ball and socket joint) is what most of us think of as the shoulder joint. This joint rolls and glides, meaning the ball (humeral head) rolls and glides downward in the socket (shoulder labrum and *glenoid fossa*) as the arm lifts overhead. The rotator cuff muscles work together to glide the humeral head downward, and if they are weak or imbalanced this can result in impingement. Another very important joint that can contribute to impingement is the scapulothoracic joint (scapular gliding along the rib cage). If someone has tight pectoralis muscles, tight upper traps, or weakness in the lower trap this can contribute to poor mobility and rhythm of the scapulothoracic joint, causing impingement.

What are some of the most common shoulder problems? Are most of them due to repetitive activities?

The most common problems I see are bicep tendonitis, impingement, frozen shoulder, bursitis, rotator cuff injury, and SLAP (Superior, Lateral, Anterior, Posterior) lesion. Adding "-itis" to the end of tendon or bursa means inflammation, which can be the cause of repetitive activities or overuse injuries. Impingement is likely associated with poor postural and imbalanced musculature. Frozen shoulder usually occurs following an injury or surgery and has more to do with the capsule (which does not contract) than musculature. Rotator cuff injuries can be from repetitive activities, from heavy lifting overhead, or even from aging tendons. SLAP lesion is usually seen in athletes, specifically baseball pitchers. This is when the long head of the biceps tendon detaches from the capsule.

For a video to help open your shoulders, visit
http://www.yogaistherapy.com/shoulder-opening-series/
All you need is a yoga strap.

If a person sleeps on their side, what arm position best supports good shoulder health? It feels like the bottom shoulder gets crunched in a side sleeping position.

I usually recommend resting more on the scapula and less directly on the side of the shoulder. The pointy and sometimes tender area on the outside of your shoulder is the acromion. When one rests directly on their side they are resting directly on the acromion, near the subacromion bursa and the supraspinatus tendon, which can be uncomfortable. What I usually recommend is resting on your side and then reaching your bottom arm in front of you so much so that your shoulder comes out from underneath you, rounding forward. When you do this you should feel the pressure more on the back side of your shoulder and shoulder blades.

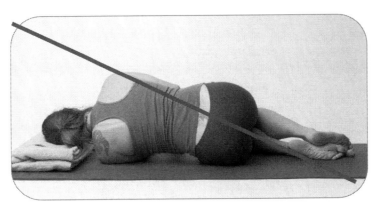

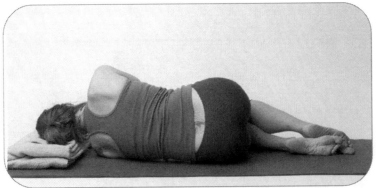

What does protraction vs. retraction of the shoulders mean, and when are these actions safely used in yoga poses?

First let's talk about the shoulder joint in more detail.

Four joints of the shoulder:

> *Clavicle: collar bone*
> *Scapula: Shoulder blade*
> *Gleno: end of the scapula that connects to the humeral head*
> *Thoracic: mid back, the vertebrae that attach to the ribs*

1. AC or acromioclavicular joint: very little movement, meant for stability, connects the clavicle (collar bone) to shoulder blade

2. SC or sternoclavicular joint: very little movement, meant for stability, connects the clavicle (collar bone) to the sternum.

3. Scapulathoracic joint: requires stability and awareness to keep shoulder joint safe, muscular connection from scapula (shoulder blade) to rib cage.

4. Glenohumeral joint: ball and socket joint, many movements, requires stability of the three other joints to move safely.

Protraction is an action of the scapulothoracic joint and involves the scapulae moving away from the midline (abduction) and moving towards the outer edges of the rib cage. This action is accompanied with thoracic spine flexion and shoulder internal rotation or rounding forward. Retraction is an action of the scapulae moving toward each other (midline).

This action is accompanied by thoracic spine extension and shoulder external rotation (moving towards the back of the body). It is likely that you have heard more about retraction than protraction in public yoga classes. You may hear something along the lines of "squeeze your shoulder blades onto your back," and the question I often ask is "when are the shoulder blades off your back?" The scapula can wing off the back when the muscles that protract the scapula are weak. This can be seen when a person is in plank pose. This winging of the scapulae can strain the muscles of the rotator cuff because the rotator cuff muscles originate on the scapula. If the scapula is not connected to the rib cage this leads to instability in the one of the main shoulder joints (scapulathoracic joint). Also, the muscles surrounding the glenohumeral joint are asked to stabilize while keeping mobility in the shoulder joint. These compensations in the shoulder joint can lead to tendonitis, tightness in the upper traps and pectoralis muscles, and rotator cuff tears or strains.

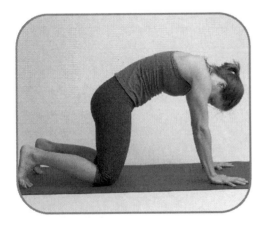 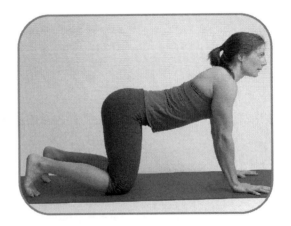

I recommend cueing your students to retract their scapulae in shoulder opening poses that also ask for the spine to move into extension, like backbends or bridge pose with fingers interlaced underneath you. I would *not* recommend cueing retraction in poses where the upper body is weight bearing, like plank, down dog, half plank, or side plank. I would instead cue protraction to assure the scapula musculature is engaged, specifically the *serrantus anterior* to keep the scapula connected to the rib cage. I recommend teaching students to feel their shoulder blade muscles.

What precautions should be taken for students with rotator cuff injuries?

The rotator cuff creates a cuff around the head of the humerus bone (upper arm bone) and is made up of four muscles: the *supraspinatus, infraspinatus, teres minor,* and *subscapularis.*

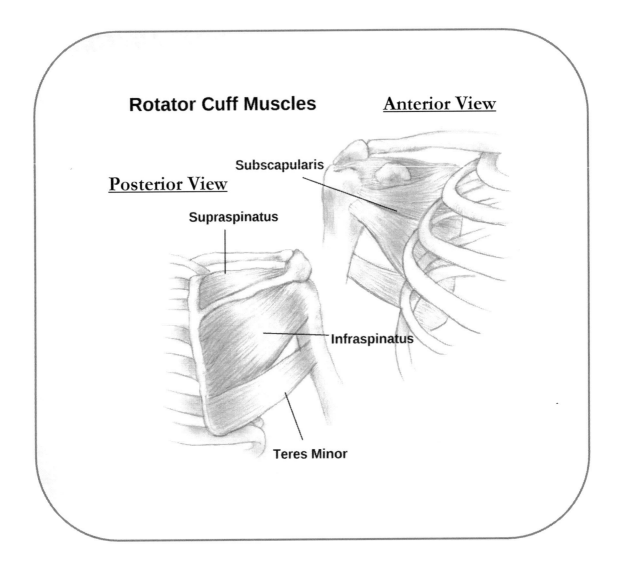

The muscle bellies of the rotator cuff muscles originate on the scapula and insert around the top and sides of the humerus. The rotator cuff muscles work together to glide the humerus downward in order to avoid the humerus contacting the acromion process of the scapula. The tendon of the supraspinatus runs underneath the acromion. If the rotator cuff muscles are weak or compromised, this can cause impingement syndrome which causes pain on the outside of the shoulder. Students who have rotator cuff injuries tend to have difficulty and pain when raising their arm up overhead. I would recommend having students with rotator cuff injuries work in "hand and knees" position and work with scapular stability (see information on page 101). I would also recommend having the student raise his/her arms in a scaption plane which is 45 degrees in front, like he/she were carrying a big beach ball and lifting it overhead. This scaption angle is said to align the scapula and the humerus in the same plane. I have students perform this with their thumbs up. If the student's ability to participate in yoga is significantly limited, I would recommend having him/her see a healthcare professional. Also remember it is possible for a student to have a rotator cuff injury or tear and still have full strength and function. Rotator cuff muscles, like joints, skin, and hair, change as we age and can degenerate but they don't necessarily cause pain or limitations.

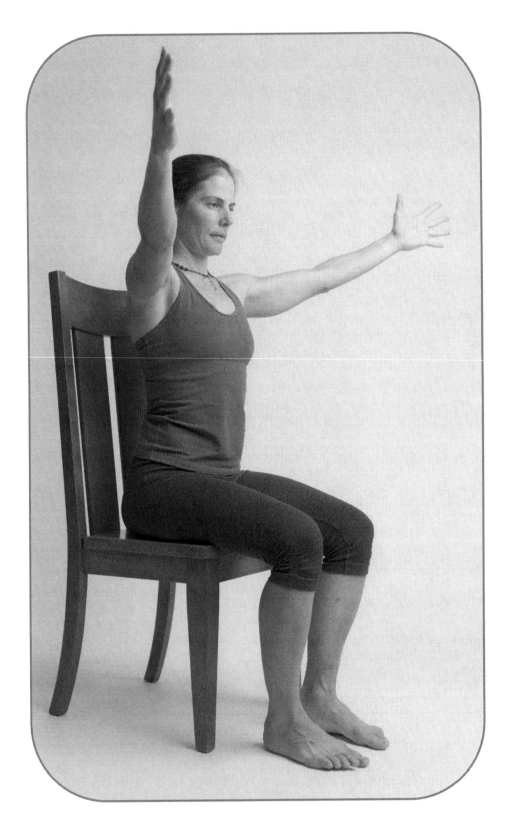

The scaption plane for the shoulders

What actions can help you feel your shoulder blade muscles?

The shoulder blade (scapulothoracic joint) moves in six different directions along the rib cage like the glenohumeral (ball and socket shoulder joint): elevation, depression, upward rotation, downward rotation, retraction, and protraction. The important fact to know about the shoulder blade is that it is where all the rotator cuff muscles originate, therefore, it is important to bring awareness and stability to this area. One of the best ways to feel this connection is in "hands and knees" position, like you are preparing to do cat and cow pose. Start first with spreading your fingers and finding whether you prefer pointing your index finger, middle fingers or thumb webbing straight ahead. Align your elbow pits with your thumb and keep the elbow pits steady and elbows straight throughout this exercise.

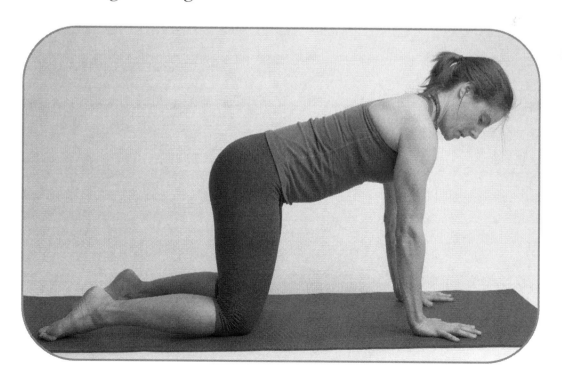

The goal of these exercises is to connect the actions in your hands to your shoulder blades. Start by pushing your hands straight down like you are pushing your hands through the ground. Feel the shoulder blade spread on your back. This action is called protraction. Protraction helps keep the shoulder blades connected to the rib cage by a muscle called the *serrantus anterior*. Then, pull your hands apart like you are trying to pull the mat apart into a right and left side, and finally pull your hands back towards your knees to connect your arms to your torso. All of these actions are done with your hands "glued" to the mat and are isometric contractions of the shoulder blade stabilizing muscles. Now try to do all three actions at the same time: Press your hands down, apart, and back. *Breathe.* I use this technique whenever my hands are on the ground in yoga poses, and especially with the transition from down dog to plank.

Notice your transitions between poses and even in everyday life. Take time to be present during the transitions.

If I recall correctly, as we did side plank, you recommended aligning the eye of the elbow with the thumb. Is this also generally the best alignment for most people in down dog as well?

First I want to make sure that no one is teaching or doing side plank with the wrist, elbow, and shoulder stacked. Stacking the wrist, elbow, and shoulder creates compression in the shoulder joint and doesn't allow a person to push down and away to stabilize the scapula. I would recommend having the weight bearing arm be at a diagonal to allow for the student to push their hand down (into the ground) and forward.

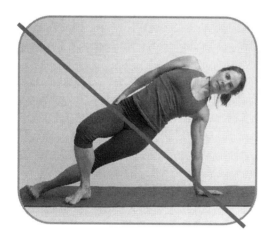 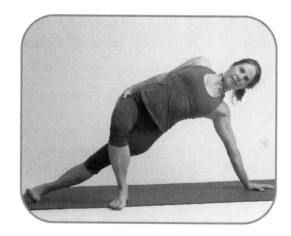

So to bring everyone on the same page, in the fourth class of my Total Back Care series, I advised about half of the class not to turn their elbow pits forward (external rotation of the shoulder) and recommended that instead they have their elbow pit aligned with their thumb.

For those of you not familiar with the term "elbow pit," it is the front side of your elbow (the opposite of the pointy side of the elbow) or the area where the nurse goes to draw blood from your arm (its official name is *antecubital fossa*). When the arms are straight, the movement of the elbow pit is a reflection of what is happening in the shoulder. When you rotate your elbow pit forward you are externally rotating the humerus (upper arm bone) and supinating the forearm. This action can help open up the shoulder and clear the tendon (long head of the biceps) from being pinched in the front of the shoulder. It can also help straighten the elbow fully which is a stable position for a portion of the elbow joint.

The elbow joint involves the connection of three bones: the ulna, radius, and humerus. We often identify the elbow as the ulnohumeral joint (tip of the elbow). However, there is another joint called the radioulnar joint which is the connection of the radial head and ulna. The radial head is important because it moves when a person supinates (palm up) or pronates (palm down) the forearm.

Find the "good enough" point in your yoga pose.
Find the balance of effort and relaxation.
Find the position where you are still able to breathe deeply and calmly through your nose.

When I asked my students to align their elbow pit with their thumb, I noticed that they very easily supinated and externally rotated the arm. A student who is able to do this easily is at risk for hyperextending their elbow and disrupting the weight distribution through their elbow and shoulders.

As you can see in the picture below, this person has hypermobility in her elbows. This causes her elbows to move inward (medially) and disturbs the stability in her elbows and shoulders, creating more pressure on the front and inside of the shoulder, the very area we are trying to keep open with external rotation.

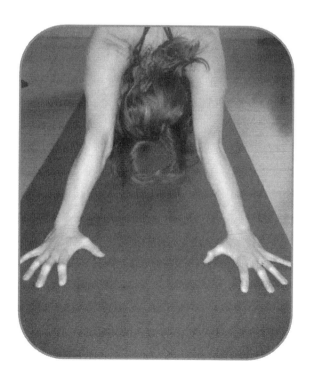
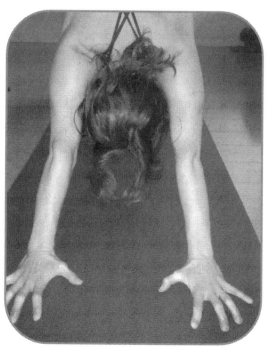

Imagine you were building a structure that would carry the weight of the body. You would want a straight line versus a line with a slight bow in it. In the picture to the right on the previous page, you can see she brings her elbow pits more towards facing each other, which brings her elbows to a straight position without hyperextension. This always allows her biceps to engage and stabilize the front of her shoulder. She noted her shoulder felt stronger and more stable when the elbow pits faced in more.

How do you know if you should rotate your elbow pits out or not?

As I indicated above, if your elbow tends to hyperextend easily or your elbow pits rotate almost without your control then I would recommend bringing your elbow pit at about a 45 degree angle, or aligned with your thumb, and then see how this feels in your shoulders. For some people who have a large carrying angle (the angle between the humerus and the forearm) or are really hypermobile in their elbows, I recommend keeping elbow pits facing each other as long as they don't have pain or pinching in the front of their shoulder.

Who should rotate their elbow pits outward?

Students who have tight shoulders find rotating the elbow pits out to be a challenge. Although opening the shoulders tends to be a focus of a lot of yoga classes, it is also equally as important to keep stability in the shoulder especially when weight bearing on one or both arms. Muscle tightness in the shoulders tends to originate from the pectoralis muscles (which internally rotate, flex and adduct the arm). They tend to be tighter and stronger than the external rotators (rotator cuff muscles). I would be cautious with overly rotating the elbow pits forward if you have a history of rotator cuff injury or shoulder issues so that you may avoid straining the rotator cuff muscles.

Like many cues in a public yoga class, this is a generalized statement for a large group of students. Ultimately, you have to figure out what feels safest and best for you and your shoulders and elbows. Try to feel a connection from your hand all the way up to your shoulder blade. What actions help you feel strong, stable, and open in your shoulders?

Do something outside of your comfort zone.
Try a new yoga class or place yourself in a situation that may be outside of your comfort zone.
Watch your breath and keep your breath calm and deep.

What do you think about "wild thing"? Am I ruining my student's shoulders?

I have received this question from a handful of yoga teachers after they read an article stating that "wild thing is unable to be done safely without potentially harming the shoulder". I have taken only a few statements from this article to explain and answer this question.

So let's first start by talking about what "wild thing" is. "Wild thing" is technically an arm balance, with one hand on the ground, both feet on the ground, and one arm reaching overhead and towards the ground. The pose is performed from down dog or side plank, and involves rotating the rib cage and pelvis up towards the ceiling and pivoting the upper body on the weight bearing arm. This pose is not recommended for beginner yoga students, and I do agree there are definitely risks involved. I was asked by a few teachers if I teach this pose and the answer is no. However, I do practice this pose.

Read Matthew Remski's full article on wild thing:

http://matthewremski.com/wordpress/tag/wild-thing/

Here is Matthew Remski's 2014 statement on wild thing, quoted from his blog *Matthew Remski: Writing, Yoga, Ayurveda.*:

> *If, as the yogi goes into the backbend, the scapula is not protracted and depressed and the humerus is not externally rotated, the head of the humerus will smash into the acromium process and create impingement and/or a tear or fraying of the supraspinatus. Doing all three of these things successfully in this scenario is next to impossible for the average yoga practitioner.*

In my words, he is suggesting that in order for the scapula (shoulder blade) to be stable and the shoulder to be safe, the scapula needs to be away from the spine and pulled down away from the ear. The humerus (arm bone) needs to be rotated outward (elbow pit towards the front). The acromium is a part of the scapula that hooks over the top of the humerus. It is considered the point of the shoulder and the supraspinatus tendon (one of the rotator cuff muscles) runs between the acromium and the humeral head. Symptoms of impingement or tearing/fraying of the supraspinatus are pain or tenderness on the outside of the arm near the deltoid along with pain or tenderness while moving the arms out to the side and up overhead. The supraspinatus lies underneath the deltoid and helps initiate abduction (bringing the arm out to the side). I do agree that it would be a challenge to keep protraction and depression of the scapula along with humeral external rotation while doing "wild thing".

To quote Reminski again,

> *If the yogi goes further into wild thing, my interviewee explained, things get worse. To bring that top foot behind the supporting leg and incrementally increase the spinal extension just doubles down on the shoulder torture, especially given that the scapular elevation associated with the full beauty of the pose (drawing the scapula up beyond the top ribs) will tend to turn off the serratus anterior. My subject's analysis concluded that the pose is destabilizing by definition to the shoulder joint, and that it can only really be approached by very flexible people who would derive no benefit from it. It cannot help but to wear out the shoulder.*

Spine extension is bringing the mid-back into a backbend which would create retraction (scapula drawing in towards the spine). Retraction of the scapula inhibits the serrantus anterior muscle which protracts the scapula and keeps the scapula connected to the rib cage (creating stability in the shoulder).

So to answer the question, "is wild thing safe to teach," my answer is, as always, it depends. I try my best not to absolute about anything because there is likely another side to the story.

- Is wild thing a risky pose for the shoulder? For sure.
- Can it be done more safely? I believe so.

Most injuries in yoga happen during the transition into or out of the pose. Transition into and out of "wild thing" is tricky and complicated.

My recommendation, if you are going to continue to teach wild thing, is to make the elbow pit point towards the thumb and keep the humerus (arm) steady. Don't let it move internally or externally, and keep the hand in front of the shoulder (not directly underneath it). And, if you need to rotate the arm outward more then move the hand instead of the humerus. I would also recommend pushing your planted hand down and forward to shift the weight more into the feet than the hand. Also pull your heel towards your hand to engage your hamstrings. Doing this will help keep you from using your quadriceps (pushing your feet forward) which will shift weight into your single hand on the ground. I would **NOT** recommend any student who has shoulder pain, history of rotator cuff tear or injury to perform this pose. One of the reasons I do not teach this pose is because many students have a history of shoulder pain, surgeries, or injuries.

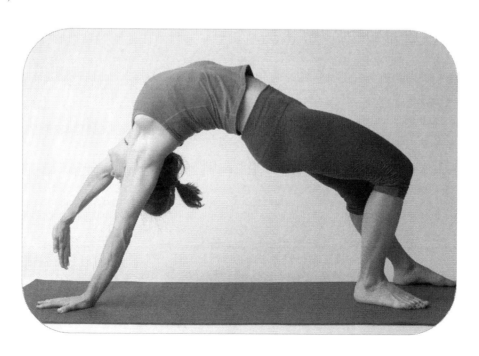

Regarding bridge pose, do we tuck the tail/pelvic tilt to connect the lower back to the earth then lift up, or no tuck/tilt? I have heard and even taught it both ways and I'm still not sure what is best. What do you think?

I believe it depends on the person and direction and purpose of the pose. I need to first say I am not a fan of the term "tuck the tailbone" for a few reasons:

1. The only muscles that attach to the tailbone are the pelvic floor muscles, which most students are not aware of, or have no idea how to access.

2. Students often squeeze their glutes and thrust their pelvis forward when asked to tuck their tailbone.

3. I like to have students touch the area I am talking about, and I find the tailbone quite personal for students to find. Instead of saying "tucking the tailbone", I prefer to cue from the area where the muscles are located which contribute to posterior tilting of the pelvis.

I speak instead of the pubis bone or *pubis symphysis* which is located on the front of pelvis. I often instruct students to pull the pubic bone forward and up if I want them to do a similar act to tucking their tail. The muscle that attaches to the pubic bone is the *rectus abdominus* and it helps to create a posterior tilt or tucking of the pelvis.

The contraction of the *rectus abdominus* during backbends is thought to help create a more universal curve in the low back and helps avoid a hinging at the most flexible lumbar section. When backbending the pelvis moves anteriorly (opposite of tucking), the lumbar spine moves into extension along (to a lesser degree) with the thoracic and cervical spine. Backbends occur primarily in the lumbar spine and the cue to tuck your tailbone is to keep students from "dumping into" (hyperextending) their low back. I would first recommend to stop talking about the tailbone and instead talk about the actions of the legs and abdominals. When a student is doing bridge pose I would recommend for him/her to use his/her hamstrings to help him/her lift his/her hips. Engaging their hamstrings will help connect him/her to their abdominal muscles. This will help your student find the muscles that will help him/her in the pose as opposed to telling him/her where his/her tailbone should or shouldn't be.

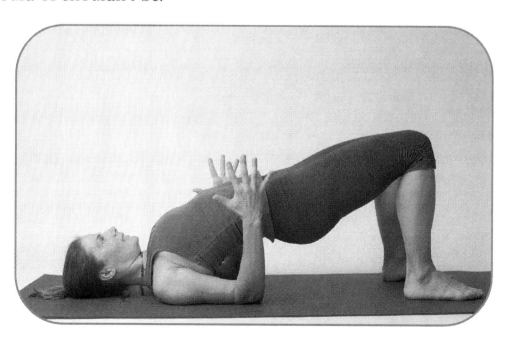

I did reverse bow (wheel pose) for the first time even though I didn't really think I'd even get up so I went for it. I had no idea what I looked like or what the arm placement was like. I just remember everyone in class telling me "you are doing it!" I felt a cramp in my right shoulder and knew I needed to get out and I had help coming down slowly. Now my shoulder is sore and I plan to rest and do light stretching. Do you have any ideas on how I might do better next time? Or should I never try it again?

I can relate to being in a class and deciding to do a pose beyond what I thought I can do. I have noticed this challenge even more since I have been on a backbend break. Although having encouragement from your classmates is helpful it may also feed into pushing yourself beyond what is safe in your body. I remind my students that yoga is about breath and movement and the breath is the priority. My first question is, "Were you breathing while you were in the pose?" If your answer is "I don't know" or "No," then I would recommend practicing different stages of the pose and making sure you can breathe in each stage.

To see a technique I use to help teach and prepare for wheel pose, visit http://www.yogaistherapy.com/preparation-for-wheel-pose/

I am not sure you should take wheel completely off your wish list for yoga poses. I would recommend opening certain areas of your body before attempting it again. Since a lot of functional activities are done with our attention in front of us, the front of the body, including hip flexors, abdominals, and shoulder muscles (pecs) tend to be shorter. When doing a backbend, especially wheel, the front of the body is being lengthened. It is quite common for students to injure their shoulder and low back trying to do a deep back bend because it usually takes more than just one yoga class to lengthen the front of the body enough to do backbends.

I would also recommend having your teacher help you next time you attempt to come up in wheel. Assure you have stretched the front of the hips and shoulders and prepared the back of your body with your belly down for back bends like cobra and *shalabasana*.

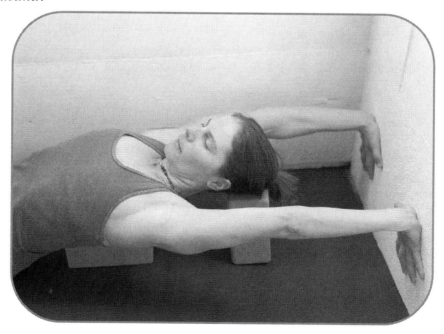

three: posture & spine

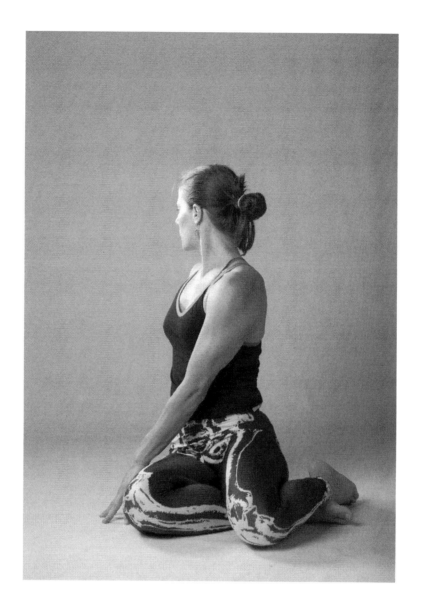

The spine is the center axis of the body and yoga helps to bring strength, mobility, and ease to the spine. This next series will address questions regarding the spine starting from the head to the tailbone.

What yoga poses can help TMJ? Can "Lion's Breath" help?

This is a great question. TMJ stands for temporomandibular joint. "TMJ" is not technically a diagnosis but is often used as a description of having a problem in your jaw. People often say, "I have TMJ," to which the know-it-all side of me wants to say, "We all have TMJ!" However, I understand that this translates to a person having a TMJ disorder or pain.

The TMJ is the hinge joint of the jaw and is the connection between the mandible (what we think of as the jaw) to the temporal bone (the cheek bone, which is part of the skull). You can feel your TMJ moving by sticking your little fingers in your ears, moving them towards your nose and opening and closing your jaw. This joint helps us chew, yawn, and talk. So needless to say it is used all the time. There is a disc between the two joint surfaces which provides a cushion for the joint.

There are two main temporomandibular disorders (TMD) caused from either 1) tightness or 2) laxity in the joint. I have found that most students have tightness from clenching or grinding their teeth. Stress is the leading cause of clenching and grinding. The disc can dislocate secondary to ligament laxity which can cause the jaw to lock in the open position. There are several causes for TMD, including trauma, poor posture, and holding the mouth open for too long.

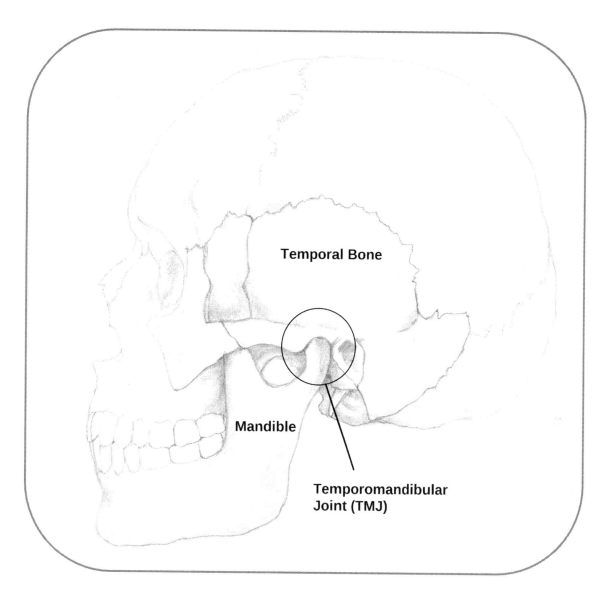

The TMJ is very closely related and influenced by the neck. When someone's head is significantly forward and their chin is tilted upwards, their TMJ can be compressed. One of the most important techniques in working with students with TMJ is addressing their head and neck position. The mandible (jaw bone) should be perpendicular to the ground with the ears directly over the shoulders and shoulders resting down away from ears. It is important to try to keep a natural concave curve in the neck without lifting the chin.

I find this easiest to attain by placing my hand on the back of my neck as I bring my ears over my shoulder and keep my chin parallel to the ground. This technique can be used in all your yoga poses, especially with back bends.

Another important technique is to notice when you are clenching your teeth. I find a good way to keep from clenching is to place the tip of my tongue behind my front top teeth where the gums and teeth connect. This helps bring the jaw to a more relaxed and neutral position that makes clenching the teeth much more difficult. I do think "lion's breath" can be helpful for students with tightness; however, I would recommend caution to any student who has a history of their jaw locking or disc dislocating with their mouth opened wide. I feel all yoga poses can be beneficial for TMD when there is awareness in the head and neck position throughout one's practice and awareness when one is clenching the teeth. I feel one of the most powerful tools yoga gives us is an opportunity to observe our bodies and our reactions to stress within our bodies.

---

*If you find yourself clenching your jaw,
take your tongue to the back of your top front teeth
and let your jaw hang and relax (separate your teeth).
Take 10 deep breaths.*

Can yoga be good for whiplash?

Whiplash can be a bit tricky to work with depending on the cause and how long symptoms have been present. I would first recommend starting with diaphragmatic breathing and releasing the pectoralis muscles (see video link on page 79). When someone sustains whiplash, his/her neck muscles are usually very tight and in protection mode. I would be cautious with stretching or a pose where the neck is unsupported and the arms are lifted like Warrior 2 pose. Instead, work with poses with his/her head supported on the ground and small roll underneath his/her neck to help encourage a neutral concave curve in the neck. Standing poses can be performed with his/her back to the wall and placing a thin block behind his/her head to give his/her support and stability for the neck. I would work with isometric movements in all planes including forward/back (flexion/extension), side bending, and rotation. I would also recommend teaching students to place the tip of their tongue to the back of their top front teeth, as this can help them keep a neutral position in their jaw and keep them from clenching their jaw.

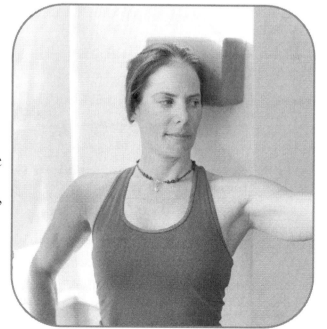

Why do we cause pain when trying to release and relax our psoas?

The psoas is active any time we are standing and walking, and even has to sustain a contraction while sitting for long periods of time. It is also a muscle that is commonly tight when we are stressed or have stimulated the sympathetic nervous system because it wants to help get it us out of danger by fighting, freezing, or fleeing.

> The sympathetic nervous system is part of the autonomic nervous system. When the sympathetic nervous system is stimulated muscles including the psoas and other hip flexors tighten to prepare the body to fight, flight, or freeze. This can happen when we experience a physical threat like someone rear-ending us or if we sit and stress for a living.

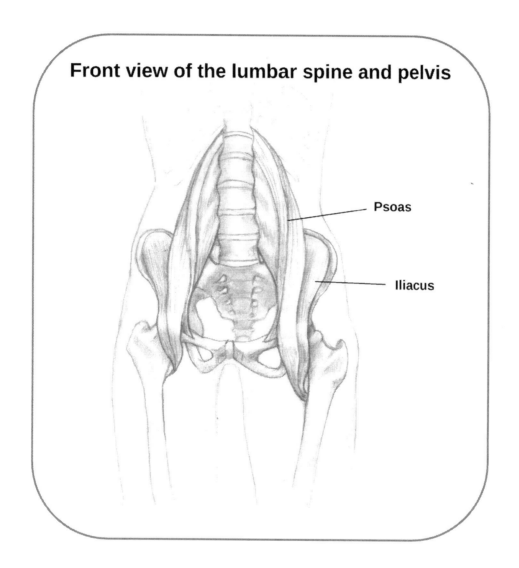

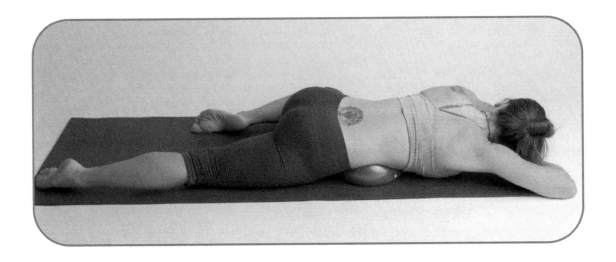

In my "So what about your Psoas" classes I have my students use a deflated ball or block to add pressure to the psoas, which can be very uncomfortable. This technique of using pressure to release a muscle is called trigger point release and is thought to help reset the muscle spindle and release the relentless contraction of the muscle. The psoas gets most restricted and stiff from sitting for long periods of times with limited movement. When one moves the body out of the psoas' sustained position, such as standing, it may result in pain in the low back or hip area. Palpating the psoas is tricky because it is located deep within the belly. Most people know they have found it because it is tender when palpated which is likely from it being stiff and tight. When steady, sustained pressure is added to the psoas muscle along with deep relaxing breathing, the psoas will likely release and soften after a few minutes.

I would not recommend this release to be performed while menstruating or pregnant or with anyone who has had recent abdominal or spinal surgery.

It is not uncommon to have some soreness after releasing your psoas. Unfortunately, the body is unable to determine the difference from good pain (to release) and bad pain (injury). In this practice of yoga, it is important to recognize when we are hurting ourselves and when we are producing discomfort for a positive result. Ultimately, we always have the ability to stop any discomfort that arises in our bodies by releasing the position. We also have the ability to choose whether to react to this discomfort or not. It is important that we trust the teacher, practitioner, or ourselves when feeling discomfort. It is a good idea to explore why this discomfort is ok and at what point it is causing harmful effects to our bodies.

> *Take time to talk to your pain.*
> *It may seem silly, but keep it simple.*
> *Ask your pain, "What would you like?"*
> *(much like trying to figure out*
> *how to help a crying child)*

What is the best treatment for low back pain? Is ice or heat better?

The rule of thumb for acute injuries is RICE: Rest, Ice, Compression, Elevation. This works well for ankle and knee injuries as well because this technique reduces inflammation, which leads to swelling and pain. However, when you are talking about low back pain, ice can help with the inflammation, but can also lead to tightening of back muscles and result in increased pain. I personally recommend castor oil either directly on the skin or saturated on a cloth with a heating pad. Please be aware castor oil will leave oil residue on any fabric it touches. Some people use plastic wrap around the castor oil pack to protect their clothing. I also highly recommend Epson salt baths for 15-20 minutes in warm water.

Regarding ice vs. heat, this depends on whether your injury or pain is a result of muscle tightness or joint inflammation. As stated above, ice relieves inflammation but tightens muscles, so if your pain is focused in the SI area or another bony area of your body, you may find relief with ice. If you find your back muscles are very tight with spasms, I would recommend heat to the area, specifically, if your pain tends to be along the erector spinae muscles (the railroad track like musculature located on either side of your spine).

Whether you choose heat or ice, it is important to check the skin within ten to fifteen minutes of use to assure there is no blistering, burning, or frost bite. It is also important to use a towel or sheet between the ice or heat source to protect your skin from overexposure. Heat can be applied up to several hours, but ice should be applied to the area for only fifteen minutes and then taken off to thaw out. If ice is applied greater than fifteen minutes, your body starts bringing blood flow back to the area as a survival response to avoid freezing. This is the opposite of what you want the ice to do. Ultimately, your body will let you know which source, heat or ice, works best for you.

> *Before saying "yes" to another party*
> *or going back for another helping of food or another drink,*
> *pause and take three deep breaths. Then ask yourself,*
> *"Does this serve me?"*

I had a really difficult time with my back when I started my yoga practice. You explaining the need to keep the natural curve of the lumbar section really helped. My back actually does feel better overall. But when I lay down on my back, legs bent or straight, there seems to be tension that I need to release. I try to get to my yoga classes a few minutes early to just lay down and let the tension melt, but I experience the same problem when I go to bed at night. When I'm up and moving around, there's no problem, but when I initially lie down, there's pain. This is only in the lumbar area above the sacrum. Why is this, and is there anything I can do about it?

Usually we feel our discomforts most when we are at rest because we aren't distracted and are more present and aware of our bodies in the resting state. I imagine your low back muscles may be transitioning from "go mode" or "on mode" to "resting mode" which may cause discomfort from change in blood flow and muscle tension to the area. Resting flat on our backs can also place muscles that (are engaged to) keep us upright (like hip flexors and back extensors) in a stretched or released state, which is almost completely the opposite of being upright.

I would recommend resting on your side for a few minutes before turning to lay flat on your back. While resting on your side, place a pillow between your knees and ankles to support your lower body. Then after two to three minutes, roll onto your back. This will help make your transition from standing or sitting to resting on your back an easier transition for your hip and back muscles.

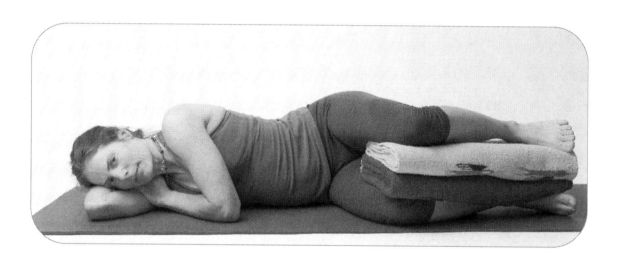

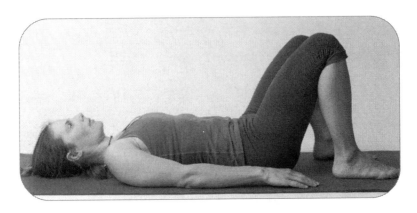

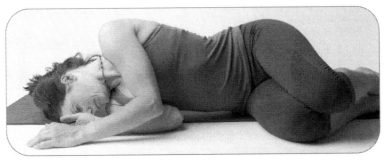

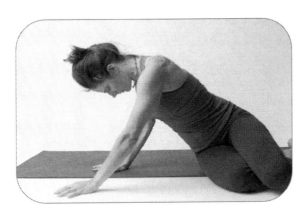

I recommend this technique anytime you transition from laying down to sitting or standing up, and/or on or off your mat: First roll onto your side. When you are getting up from bed, let your feet come down towards the ground. Finally, use your arms to sit up.

This may seem like it will take longer than just sitting up. However, after a few times, it is just as quick and much better for your body.

How do I know if I have good posture?

When we are talking about good posture we are talking about maintaining the slight "s" shape of our spine. Our postures change as we move. The general rule with posture is to maintain proper spinal alignment and curves while performing activity or sustain postures, like standing or sitting for long periods of time. Posture starts from your feet and your pelvic alignment. A good starting place is to look down at your feet, while you are sitting or standing, and to assure your feet are pointing straight ahead. More specifically, your second toe should be pointing straight ahead. Then look at your knee caps and assure they are pointing straight ahead. The pelvic alignment can be a bit tricky. If you place your hand on the boney area of your hips and tilt your pelvis slightly forward (think of your pelvis as a bowl pouring water out onto your feet) this will help bring a slight curve to your low back (lordosis). Moving up to your shoulder, gently pull the bottom tips of shoulder blades down towards your hips and towards each other. Also rotate the palms of your hands and biceps forward, this is called external rotation of the shoulder and naturally decreases the rounding of the shoulders. Be aware to keep a kyphotic (convex) curve in the mid-back and not to squeeze your shoulder blades too close together on your back. Last but not least, check your head and neck; place your hand on the underside of your jaw bone (mandible) and ensure that your jaw bone is parallel to the ground and then bring your head back so it is aligned between your shoulders. Take a few breaths in this "new posture" and practice throughout your day especially with sustained positions like standing washing dishes or driving in your car. It is likely that this new awareness of your posture will be challenging at first, but will get easier as your postural awareness becomes more natural.

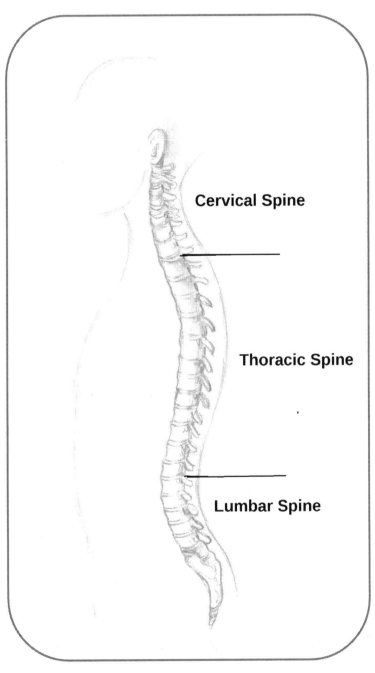

What does it mean to "lay flat on your back"?

This term is used quite a bit during yoga class and, just to clear the air, the back is not flat. What I would recommend is to check in to see that while lying on your back you can maintain the spinal curvature discussed above. To assure good posture while resting on your back, start like we did above. Making sure your feet and knee caps are pointing straight up towards the ceiling, press the lower part of your spine (just above your sacrum) down towards the ground to create a gentle curve. See if you can slide your hand underneath your low back and allow your shoulder blades to rest on the ground. Don't press your shoulders back. Check your jaw bone and assure it is perpendicular to the ground. Place your hand between your neck/head assuring there is a gentle curve. These curves may be hard to maintain when your knees are straight, so you may need to bend your knees and place your feet on the ground. Having your knees bend while resting on your back is appropriate if you have pain in your back when your knees are straight, or if you have difficulty maintaining the spinal curves. So to answer your question regarding lying flat on your back, the better term may be: "lay on your back while maintaining a slight S-curve in your spine."

I met you at Tubac Healing Arts for the teacher training program and am finally certified! I have found a small population of people interested, yet hesitant, about taking yoga because they have rods in their backs. I would love to help spread the love of the spine through yoga to these people. Do you have any recommendations?

The location of your students' spinal rods will determine where they need to be cautious. The caution with working with students with spinal rods is more for that of the area above and/or below where the rods are located. Since the space that has the rods is immobilized (not movable), the areas above and/or below will try to make up for motions that are lost. This can cause increased wear and tear on the vertebrae which may cause more pain and potential surgical intervention. If a student has spinal rods in their cervical (neck) spine then I would be cautious with headstand, shoulder stand, and extreme neck positions like fish pose. If a student has rods in their thoracic spine (mid-back/rib cage), I would be cautious with twists and chest openers. If a student has rods in their lumbar spine (low back), I would be cautious with back bends and forward bends. Students who have rods in their spine should continue their yoga practice with modifications. There will be poses that will not be safe nor possible for students to do. Keep in mind having a rod in the spine and having a spinal fusion are generally the same thing.

I find most of my students with spinal issues have lumbar or low back rods/fusions. I still have them do a modified version of cobra, in which they do all the work (i.e. pull hands back, pull top of head forward, reach toes back, and only lift their forehead off the ground while keeping everything engaged, with breath flowing deeply and calmly all the while). I would recommend focusing on increasing motion in the hips and shoulders and educating your students about breathing into the low belly and low back.

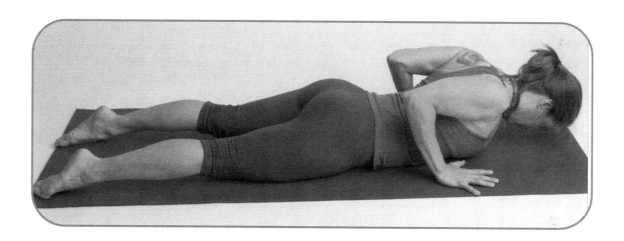

For a demonstration on how to modify cobra pose, visit
http://www.yogaistherapy.com/cobra-for-students-with-spinal-fusions/

Can imbalances in my pelvis cause chronic neck pain?

Yes, I consider the pelvis to be the foundation of the body. When the pelvis is out of alignment, which can happen from a sudden injury or cumulative habits or positioning, pain and discomfort can occur throughout the spine, shoulders, and lower body. Usually when someone has chronic neck pain the focus of the treatments is on the neck musculature, reducing tension, and decreasing overall stress. This can be an effective way to treat neck pain. In my experience, I have found assessing and treating pelvic imbalances to be the most effective approach and provides more permanent relief.

What do you think about inversion tables? Are they worth it?

I receive this question a lot from clients and students. I agree with the concept of an inversion table. Hanging upside down or slightly upside down can help create space in the body. Most people who ask me about inversion tables are interested in creating space in their low back. What I don't like about inversion tables is that you are hung from your ankles. My theory is that you have to create space in your ankles, knees, and hips before the space gets to your spine. With the inversion table, you have little control over how much pull can be created. Additionally, there is the difficulty of getting in and out of it.

Have you tried? Have someone nearby when you try getting into and out of the inversion table for the first time, trust me. If you want to create space in your spine I would recommend a technique that involves two straps and a block. This will save you at least $100 and some space in your home.

> *Contraindication for inversion tables include:*
> - *Glaucoma*
> - *Recent eye surgery*
>
> *Caution with:*
> - *Uncontrolled hypertension (high blood pressure)*
> - *Hiatal hernia*

To see an alternative to an inversion table, visit
http://www.yogaistherapy.com/alternative-to-an-inversion-table/

I have heard you mention you aren't a fan of Yin Yoga. Why not?

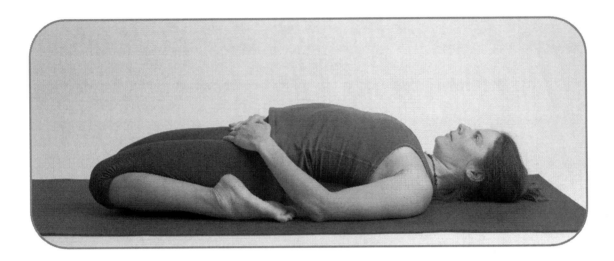

I am not a fan of yin yoga from my own experience of yin yoga. However, my relationship with yin yoga has changed in the last few years. My first experience of yin was after I just completed a six-day Anusara intensive where I was asked to stay engaged in every posture. When I was in yin yoga class the teacher keep saying let go and my body kept saying don't you dare. I did eventually let go in *supta virasana* and promptly threw out my back for a few weeks. I then revisited yin during my mentorship with my yoga teacher, Rachel Krentzman. I found it quite beneficial for my back pain, though all the poses I did were forward folds. I held the poses for two to three minutes, as opposed to five minutes. I found this practice resolved much of my low back pain. I believe my second attempt at yin was beneficial because I addressed the tightness in my low back muscles. I think yin, like many other styles of yoga including restorative, vinyasa, and power, should be done in conjunction with each other. I feel yin all by itself leads to overstretched muscles and instability which is a common condition I see in dancers and super-flexible yoga students. I have found it more challenging to teach my more flexible students about body awareness, safety, and control in yoga poses. I believe there are certain muscles including the hip flexors, piriformis, and hamstrings that need to be approached with caution to avoid aggravating low back pain, sciatica, or herniated disc. I prefer a focus on alignment while doing yin to allow the student to stay aware of his or her body during the practice.

I have a long road trip coming up and I noticed after sitting for about an hour and a half my back hurts! Are there any exercises or poses I can do that will help while I am driving or when I am a passenger?

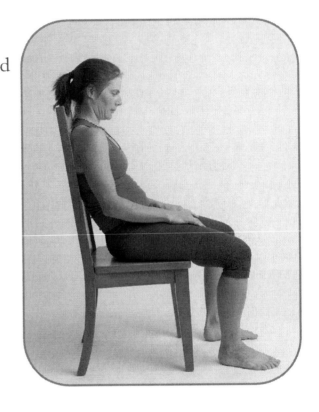

While sitting in a car for long periods of time our bodies tend to go into a relaxed mode leading to a sustained position for long periods with poor or no postural awareness. The most common position I observe and even I take while driving is a slouched posture with my knees turned out and away from each other with the pelvis curled underneath (see picture above). This causes a person to sit more on the sacrum (low part of my back) and less on the ischial tuberosities (sitting bones). This position is surprisingly comfortable while driving except after long periods of time. What this position does is overstretch your low back muscles, disengaging our legs and abdominal, and contributes to tight external rotators (including the piriformis muscle) that can lead to back pain and hip pain.

To change this position you may need to scoot your butt back into the seat and then tilt your pelvis forward slightly to allow the sitting bones/ischial tuberosities to be on the seat.

Check to see if there is a slight concave curve in your low back. Some people like to place a roll on the back of the seat to support their low back. This is a good idea as long as you use the roll to remind you to maintain a curve and not as a back rest. Once you are seated on your sitting bones, place your feet on the floor board and hug your knees toward each other so that your thighs are parallel to each other and your knees point straight ahead (see picture to right). You can pretend as though you are holding a block between your knees. Do your best to maintain this position for as long as possible while driving. Check yourself every half hour or so to see if you are maintaining a good position. Sometimes you will have to adjust your car seat and maybe even add a solid cushion on your seat to adding extra height or stability to the seat.

A few simple exercises to perform while driving to relieve discomfort in your hips, back, or glutes are: Glute squeeze, weight shifting from one buttock to another, and rotating your knees in and out. Of course taking breaks while driving to stretch your legs and walk is always a good idea.

I am traveling for the holidays and I find my body gets really tense on the plane. Do you have any stretches you would recommend to do while I am traveling so my body feels better when I arrive?

One time when I was traveling I had my "yoga is therapy" shirt on and the guy sitting next me to asked if I would teach a yoga class to the plane. Yes, I did strongly consider it. Traveling on the plane is challenging since the seats are so cramped with the limited amount of space and ability to bring props with you. Let me give you some small movements to work with.

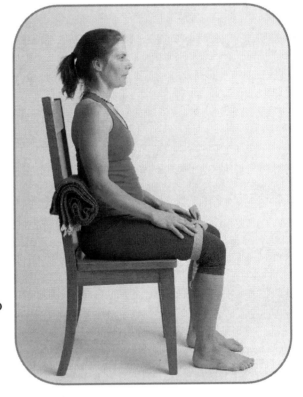

First let's talk about what might be helpful to have with you. Since you may be traveling someplace cool, you may have a sweater or jacket that you can place behind you to help maintain a concave lumbar curve. I would recommend scooting your hips all the way to the back of the seat and place the small rolled up sweater or jacket just above your hips and below your ribs. If it is too uncomfortable, consider making the roll smaller. Maybe try this at home before traveling to make sure you have a perfect size article of clothing.

Notice your thighs. Try to keep them pointing straight ahead and parallel (I do realize that if you have long legs this is next to impossible). It might be helpful to use a strap around your thighs to keep your thighs parallel. Keep your feet flat on the ground. The tendency, especially for long periods of time, is for the knees to move away from each other, the feet to roll out, and the hips to tuck underneath. This position places strain on the low back and shortens the piriformis (and other external rotators) which may cause pain and discomfort in the low back and hips. If you find yourself becoming fatigued into this position, reestablish the position above several times throughout your flight. I would also recommend pressing your knees together and walking with your feet wider than your hips (as much as you can) to help counterbalance the tendency for your knees to drift away from each other. In addition, notice if your sitting bones are even right to left, and try to evenly place your weight on each sit bone.

While in the upright and aligned position, I would recommend doing a few isometrics (engaging the muscles without moving the joint) for your hip muscles. Isometrics are great to keep blood flow to your muscles and to assist in stabilizing your joints. To engage the hamstrings (back of your legs), press your heels into the ground and pull them back (like pulling them underneath the chair). Feel the back of your legs engage but don't pull your heels away from the ground. Keep them down.

To engage your abductors (outer hips), pull your knees and feet away from each other. To engage the adductors (inner thighs) bring your feet and knees towards each other. I would recommend sustaining these contractions for 3-5 deep breaths and then release. Repeat up to ten times. If you noticed, I didn't have you engage the quadriceps (front of the thigh). There are two reasons for this. One is that your hip flexors will likely be tight from sitting so much. Engaging your quadriceps will help engage your hip flexors and create more tightness in the front of the hip. The second reason is to avoid knee pain. When the quadriceps are engaged with the knee at ninety degrees this can place a lot stress on the patella (kneecap).

For the upper body, I would recommend first making sure that if you are doing anything with your arms, like reading or typing on your computer, you have your arms supported, even if you share the armrest with your seatmate. When I travel, my upper traps (top of my shoulder) and pecs (front of the shoulder) seem to cramp up from carrying my bags. These muscles may be challenging to stretch in close quarters so I would recommend doing a release instead.

For the upper trap, place the tips of your fingers into your opposite shoulder on the meaty part between the tip of your shoulder and your neck. Press your fingers down and hold as you roll your shoulder forward and backward. Make sure to not hit the person next to you.

To release your pec muscles, take your fingertips to the opposite shoulder between your shoulder and your breast. Press your fingers in or maybe even pinch with your thumb and fingers . When releasing the pecs you may feel some numbness or tingling down the arm or hand that you are releasing. This is because you have nerves that travel underneath your pectoralis muscles. This should disappear after a minute or two of ending your release. No doubt you will find some tender spots in the top and front of your shoulders. This is normal. Try your best to keep your breath calm and deep, allowing these muscles to relax. Sustain each of these releases on each side for ten to fifteen breaths. These may be repeated as often as you would like.

The last technique I would like to recommend is "eagle arm" or "hug yourself" arm pose. Either cross your elbows with your fingers pointing up towards the ceiling ("eagle") or stack your elbows and grab the back of your shoulders ("hug yourself")

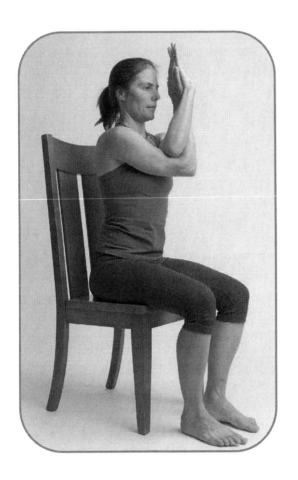
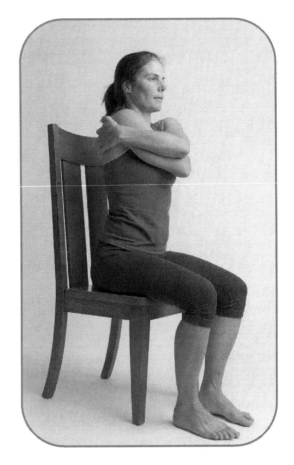

Either position is good. Bring your forehead to your hands or your chin to your chest and let your shoulder blades spread across your back. Direct your breath in between your shoulder blades and relax your neck and shoulders. Sustain for up to twenty breaths. Repeat with the other arm on top. Be careful coming into and out of pose to make sure you don't hit your seatmate.

I hope these few pointers will be helpful to release tension from your body while traveling. When in doubt, the simple act of breathing deeply will help relax your nervous system which will then relax your mind and body. I wish you safe travels.

Start a simple sitting practice.
Just sit and breathe,
or observe your thoughts.
Start with one minute and then increase
to two minutes the following week
I highly recommend using a timer.

Afterword

I recognize that there are numerous answers to the questions that were asked, some of which are very detailed and others that are much more general. Of course, my response is always determined by the clients or students I am working with. I am hoping the answers I have shared are somewhere in between, and give you enough information to understand the general concept and give you a little more information to pique your interest to investigate more.

I wish you well on your yoga journey.

Namaste,

Jaimie Perkunas, DPT e-RYT

Jaimie@yogaistherapy.com

www.yogaistherapy.com

Made in the USA
San Bernardino, CA
21 October 2016